Table of Contents

FOREWORD ....
PREAMBLE ....
INTRODUCTION ....
CHAPTER I - IF YOU WANT, YOU (
CHAPTER II - MY STORY OF CHALLENGES AND SUCCESSES 38
    WHY THIS CHAPTER? 38
    HOW MY ORDEAL BEGAN - "EPISODIC CLUSTER HEADACHE WITHOUT A PROPER DIAGNOSIS" 40
    A FEW YEARS LATER, THERE COMES THE CLUSTER HEADACHE DIAGNOSIS. 49
    THE DISTANCE BETWEEN SAYING AND DOING IS HUGE, AND DESPAIR MAKES YOU CROSS IT WITH A "LITTLE JUMP" – I DECIDE TO GO FOR SUICIDE 52
    MY EXPERIENCE IN THE HYPERBARIC CHAMBER 54
    THE DISCOVERY OF SUMATRIPTAN 56
    MY BOSS: STRESS 57
    I DON'T GIVE UP AND TRY A DIFFERENT APPROACH. 60
    BACK TO THE OLD TREATMENTS AND EARLY NON-MEDICINAL APPROACHES 61
    PRANOTHERAPY AND THE FALL OF A PILLAR - DAD'S DEATH 66
    ODD EXPERIENCES TO CONSIDER 72
    THE INFLUENCE OF EMOTIONAL SHOCKS ON CH 73
    NEW TREATMENTS AND EXPERIENCES 74
    STRANGE BUT TRUE: A CALCIUM CHANNEL BLOCKER FOR PROPHYLAXIS – VERAPAMIL 77
    A CANCER WAS ALL I NEEDED! BUT EVERY CLOUD HAS A SILVER LINING, AND I GET A NEW CONFIRMATION 79
    ARDUOUS WORK AND CH EXACERBATION - A NEW ADMISSION TO A NEW FACILITY 83
    A DREAM COMES TRUE AND THE INTERFERENCE OF EMOTIONAL SHOCKS ON CH IS CONFIRMED –O.U.C.H. Italy Onlus 86
    PERSONAL RESEARCH INTO THE COMMON TRAITS OF CH SUFFERERS 88
    TIME GOES BY AND DESPAIR MAKES ME DO ODD THINGS 92
    SOMETIMES PERSISTENCE AND COMMITMENT ARE REWARDED .. 93
    DO YOU THINK I TRIED AGAIN OR GAVE UP? 96
    OF COURSE I STILL NEED TO WORK TO EARN A LIVING 98
    PRACTICE MAKES PERFECT 99

Translated by Laura Monti – Milan (Italy)

- A NEUROLOGIST I CALL SPECIAL 101
- A CHANGE OF DIRECTION 105
- AFTER PEACE A NEW WAR 110
- CONCLUSIONS AND PEARLS OF WISDOM 115

CHAPTER III TIPS, BARRIERS, AND SOLUTIONS 121

- HABITS 122
- EMOTIONS, THOUGHTS, AND FEELINGS 126
- MAIN BARRIERS AND HOW TO OVERCOME THEM 129

CHAPTER IV MEDICATIONS 133

- VERAPAMIL 134
- CORTICOSTEROIDS - CORTISONE 137
- CARBOLITHIUM® 140
- ANTIEPILEPTICS 141
- IMIGRAN® (SUMATRIPTAN SUCCINATE 6MG SUBCUTANEOUS INJECTIONS AND 50/100MG TABLETS) 142
- OTHER MEDICATIONS AGAINST THE ATTACKS 151

CHAPTER V DRUGS 152

- PREAMBLE 152
- THC (DELTA-9 TETRAHYDROCANNABINOL) 153
- COCAINE – CODEINE 157
- PSILOCYBE – LSD – LSA 158

CHAPTER VI OXYGEN 163

CHAPTER VII THE FIRST ALLY, VERY OFTEN DISREGARDED - WATER 168

CHAPTER VIII FOOD AND FOOD SUPPLEMENTS 173

- THE KETOGENIC DIET 184

CHAPTER IX THE HOLISTIC VISION 187

- INTRODUCTION 187
- PRIMARY HEADACHE 189
- WHAT THE BEAST MEANS TO TELL US 192
- UNDERSTANDING AND INFLUENCING THE BEAST 196

FRIENDS, FAMILY, DOCTORS, SCHOLARS 211

CONCLUSION 230

DISCLAIMER 236

Translated by Laura Monti – Milan (Italy)

FOREWORD

I have known Davide and the founders of the then newborn "OUCH Italy Onlus" (Organization for Understanding Cluster Headache) for almost twenty years, since the beginning of 2000. We first spoke on the phone, met on the road, and got to know each other at a restaurant in Milan, like we usually do with friends. Riccardo and Sten, two of the OUCH Founding Members, were with him and, at the time, I was the President of AIC (*Associazione Nazionale dei Pazienti Cefalalgici*, the national association of headache patients). We knew right away that there were lots of useful things we could do together in the field of headaches.

A patient with Cluster Headache is not like any other person. Those that, like me, have to deal with these patients on a daily basis know very well that this illness does not strike at random. Davide fully confirms this not too medical, not too scientific, yet well-known fact. People with cluster headache tend to be brilliant, strong-willed, determined, deeply committed, and rich of ideas. This is exactly what I noticed when I first met Davide. Since then we have been on a journey in which we often struggled side by side to obtain institutional acknowledgements, discover new strategies to improve pain control, spread knowledge and information, and explore new ways and new treatment options. In short, we have been trying to do everything useful to improve the quality of life of these patients and make my work as a physician focused on this disorder more meaningful, both for health and for society.

Davide had an all but easy life: in addition to CH, as cluster headache is often briefly referred to, he was ravaged by other serious diseases that would have destroyed both the body and the mind of many. I was always amazed by his ability to put up even with serious diseases and to react beyond any rules and limits. But

Translated by Laura Monti – Milan (Italy)

this is Davide: an uncommon disease for a definitely uncommon person, often hostile to the rules, including those of common sense. If this had not been the case, there would obviously have been no way out for him.

This book is a testimony, not of illness – you could find plenty in any scientific book – but of determination, of a way to react, to cope with illness, to be an active player in one's own life, for better or for worse, which is almost stunning. An attitude that, I believe, does not depend on the "beast" that tormented him, but one that has an absolute value, whatever the illness. Each page tells about an unimaginable world and forces you to think. I do not know what the truth is, I am not sure there can be one in medicine. Each patient has his or her own truth, and this book contains a very peculiar, subjective, and often unexpected truth – that of Davide. It is certainly not absolute, but it is *his* truth and, as such, deserves to be listened to and respected. While I do not agree on everything you will read in this book, I respect the point of view of Davide, even if it may be difficult to understand, and even more difficult to share. I fully agree on many other aspects, though, and believe that this continuous mutual sharing of views and positions has a positive impact on the two of us.

Don't take this as blasphemy. Physicians learn from books that are often summaries, or even transfigurations of reality. What a great chance, then, to be able to learn directly from the real life of patients! Attending OUCH meetings in recent years has taught me a lot, and I trust I have been able to pass on these teachings to the benefit of all my patients.

This is why, when Davide asked me to reread and revise his book, I was more than happy to help him. In a field like that of headaches, and of cluster headache in particular, where so many speak up without having enough knowledge, where scientific "truths" are scarce, rare, and strictly measured out, and the

Translated by Laura Monti – Milan (Italy)

opinions of leaders often represent the only scientific "truth", I believe that the opinion of our patients is just as important – if not, indeed, decisive – to learn about their true way of living that reaches far beyond their medical history which, as such, is hardly capable to describe the patient's actual experience. I know that Davide has been pursuing for many years a direct and often "intimate" confrontation with other patients who, like him, suffer from cluster headache, and that his determination led him to discover common traits that lurk in the folds of the existence of a CH sufferer. I was lucky enough to discuss with him all these aspects, which can hardly come to the surface during "ordinary" neurological examinations (due to time limits).

I trust that this book will reach many physicians. They may be horrified at reading certain paragraphs but, if they are patient and humble enough to listen to the voice of suffering, they will be able to see things from a completely different point of view and to penetrate into aspects of our patients that often escape traditional communication channels. But I also trust that reading this book will provide new insights to enrich research and open up still unexplored paths.

Fabio Frediani
President, ANIRCEF
(Associazione Neurologica Italiana per la Ricerca sulle Cefalee)
Director
Headache Center - U.O.C. Neurology and Stroke Unit
S. Carlo Borromeo Hospital
ASST – Saints Paul and Charles – Milan

Milan, October 2018

PREAMBLE

Hello, my name is Davide. My full name is Davide Luca Schiantarelli, a.k.a. "Skianta," as my friends call me, and I am one of the five founding members of O.U.C.H. Italy Onlus (Organization for Understanding Cluster Headache).

My main goal in writing this book on cluster headache is to help you. Whether you are a cluster headache sufferer, a relative or a friend of a sufferer, a researcher or a physician, if you continue reading this book you will have more opportunities to move forward in your journey. By this I mean, if you are a sufferer, to manage to suffer less; if you are a friend of a sufferer, to learn some do's and don'ts to support and help a sufferer; if you are a physician, to get closer to understanding this serious disease, to be of greater help to the people you take care of, and to better guide them through many of those aspects that you often have no opportunity to explore in the limited time available for the examinations; last but not least, if you are a researcher, I trust I will be able to throw some light on still unexplored paths.

I am a technician, my job is to ensure health and safety in the construction industry. I work for Saipem, part of the ENI group. I am in charge of protecting the health of the workers so that they do not incur in accidents or develop disorders caused by

Translated by Laura Monti – Milan (Italy)

occupational diseases. I also deal with the design and provision of training programs, also in the field of safety and R&D projects.

I was married to a beautiful woman named Annalisa and I have two lovely daughters, Giada and Fiaba, who gave me the strength to continue on my difficult life journey.

Since I founded the association, to which I devoted over ten years of my life, I have been pursuing a specific goal: **understand what cluster headache is and try to beat it, or at least tame it, in order to improve the quality of my life, as well as of that of others.**

A forum for cluster sufferers[1] was created within the association thorough the skills of its first president, the late Riccardo Pentenero (a close friend of mine and the first CH sufferer I ever met). The forum is still in operation and can be found at http://www.grappolaiuto.it.

This forum was a godsend for all the new CH sufferers that logged on to it and that, in doing so, could escape their painful loneliness. From a psychological point of view, knowing, confronting with, and supporting each other truly helped many people feel better.

---

[1] Throughout the book, the author uses the colloquial term "grappolati" to refer to CH sufferers, after the Italian name of the illness "cefalea a grappolo". The English for "grappolo" is, in fact, "cluster." *(Translator's Note)*

Translated by Laura Monti – Milan (Italy)

Being public, the forum had a limit, though, namely that the people posting in it often wear a "mask", i.e. don't really disclose the truth about them. And, in fact, they don't share their most intimate and confidential information.

Being aware of this limit, I embarked on an individual process that consisted in meeting in person all the CH sufferers that joined the forum and, by going out together, talking to them, getting to know some of them more intimately, I discovered some common traits.

I was greatly surprised by the fact that, even if I went out with people I had never met before and talked about the disease we shared, we soon felt like we had known each other for a lifetime, like we had been friends all along. Getting out of the limbo of loneliness was indeed a need we all shared! In doing so, important, as well as extremely intimate and strictly confidential aspects of our life, relevant to our suffering, emerged in our conversations.

I am not a writer, so please don't blame me if the quality of this book is not what you would expect, **but rather focus basically on the content, which is the only thing you need to pick up, the only one that can help you tame your own "beast"** (as cluster headache or, briefly, CH is defined in the sufferers' jargon).

Translated by Laura Monti – Milan (Italy)

I have been a cluster headache sufferer for 30 years. At first my headache was mild and episodic, then **quickly developed into a chronic drug-resistant cluster headache that ruined my entire life –** my actual existence, my job, my friendships, my moments of leisure, my mood, my social relations, and so on and so forth!

Until some time ago, my life was just cluster headache. It raged both during the day and at night. Every moment of my life was a real concentrate of fear and suffering.

My recurring thought in everyday life was, alas, suicide as the only way out of that terrible situation. I said to myself, "when you just can't take any more of it, just kill yourself," and this incredibly helped me hold on.

I remember that, at some point in time, I was no longer able to tame the beast and was offered, as a last resort, to submit to DBS (Deep Brain Stimulation), a highly invasive method that was only available at the "Carlo Besta" Institute in Milan. DBS consists in implanting an electrode across the brain, near the hypothalamus; this electrode is then connected through a wire to a stimulator, which is applied subcutaneously near the collarbone and generates electrical impulses.

I didn't want to use this option, because I thought it would be a failure, for obvious physical reasons.

Translated by Laura Monti – Milan (Italy)

Here are the reasons. The hypothalamus is known to be electrically hyperactive in CH sufferers. Therefore, if the electrode had transferred this excess energy outside and dissipated it, I would have gone for the option, but the process was, in fact, reversed: the electrode opposed to the hyperactive hypothalamus, while also introducing more energy into the brain.

Luckily, things have changed today. My cluster headache has not disappeared completely, but has turned into something I can control, something that no longer ravages my life as it did in the past, and that no longer causes me such excruciating suffering.

It was a long and difficult journey, in some respects even fortuitous and devastating, but the point of arrival is worthy of all the efforts I have made – **as I said, my beast is now under control, my beast has been tamed!**

I am writing this book because **I have set myself a new goal, namely to place all my experience, all my suffering, all my knowledge at your disposal in order to help you undertake a process of transformation aimed at keeping your beast at bay, at making you suffer less.** I would also like to help physicians and researchers understand each other better. **There is often an unknown gap** between what the outside world sees of those that suffer from CH and what these really experience, in their

Translated by Laura Monti – Milan (Italy)

minds and hearts. **I want to manage to fill this gap,** and to do so, I have laid myself completely bare.

I can't promise you that I'm going to make you feel better – far from me to arouse false hope – but I can surely help you feel a little (or much) better. This will depend on several factors, as much as on the disease. **If you can take the reins of your beast, you can tame it like I did**. It may not be easy, you may fail several times in the process but, most importantly, you may find the strength to continue towards your transformation.

Never back down, never give up, hold on!

However, in your transformation, you should be careful not to "trip yourself" because, although you may not believe what I am telling you now, your **beast is actually *you*!** Have you ever noticed that, whenever you seem to understand something about your beast, it changes, mutates, and transforms?

In medicine, the beast is classified among neurological disorders, and is called "cluster headache". I think this is a diminishing definition, because I believe that the beast is an illness that involves multiple aspects – neurological, neuroendocrine, psychological, and emotional, the latter producing a strong impact.

It is, indeed, a migraine, because it affects, from time to time, either the right side or the left side. The attacks never involve the

Translated by Laura Monti – Milan (Italy)

whole head, and that's why it is technically a migraine (i.e. a headache, or cephalalgic pain, that involves half of the head).

Translated by Laura Monti – Milan (Italy)

INTRODUCTION

Cluster headache poses a lot of challenges. It affects few people, it is a serious problem, it is an illness about which general practitioners themselves often know too little, and an illness that, in the past, was even hardly recognized as such by specialists.

Cluster sufferers are often correctly diagnosed only after receiving many incorrect diagnoses that, sometimes, even result into them taking the wrong medications. The consequence, in most cases, is to merely intoxicate the body, thus making their headache even worse.

I met dozens of CH sufferers that told me it took a few years before they could get a correct diagnosis from a neurologist. I would like to point out that this, of course, is not because physicians are inexperienced, but because the symptoms of the disease are still scarcely known.

Luckily, this situation keeps changing and has now improved considerably. But looking back a mere ten years, it was really dreadful.

Friends, family, or co-workers often do not understand cluster headache and sometimes, when they hear you suffer and complain, they just say, "Cut it short and take an Advil®!"

Translated by Laura Monti – Milan (Italy)

CH sufferers are often misunderstood and neglected, which makes them prone to anger and isolation, emotions that feed their headache.

I remember that so many times I went out with friends in my car, perhaps to go to a disco. When an attack came I suffered so much that I decided to go home, and those that shared the car with me had to leave, too. In the long run, I was left alone because they no longer wanted to share my car for obvious reasons (I was a party-pooper).

Once diagnosed, cluster headache is a difficult beast to tame because the symptomatic medication available on the market – Imigran® 6mg vials (sumatriptan succinate, a 5HT1B-D serotonin-receptor inhibitor) – to suppress the attacks at the outset can make the disease even worse if used extensively (although there is no scientific data on the subject; this claim is based on my personal experience and on direct confrontation with many CH sufferers, but is also reported in the OUCH Italy forum).

Just think that, through the interactions we had with OUCH USA, we found that the effective dose of Imigran® to stop the attack is well below 6mg, and that a 3mg dose is enough in most cases. Imigran® in 4mg doses is, in fact, already being produced in America.

Translated by Laura Monti – Milan (Italy)

These vials are not yet available on the Italian market, where Imigran® continues to be sold in various formulas, including 6mg vials.

In this respect, OUCH posted a video in the forum to teach CH sufferers how to halve the vials of Imigran®, albeit at their own risk.

The disease is difficult to tame and, in fact, another way to deal with the symptoms is to use pure oxygen at very high flow rates (7-15 Lt/min.). However this option is very often unavailable at work or away from home. **Just think that, according to medical protocols, oxygen is denied even in hospitals** (personal experience) when you are admitted for other reasons and you get cluster headache attacks.

Oxygen dispensers sold in pharmacies often do not go beyond 7 Lt/min., and CH sufferers are forced to use (when they know and have the opportunity) dispensers that offer a flow of up to 24 Lt/min., as I did at my own expense (about 350 euros).

In many Italian regions, obtaining oxygen for cluster headache is sometimes impossible or very difficult. Consider that even neurologists tend not to prescribe it, and rather go for Imigran® (see the chapter on oxygen for details).

Translated by Laura Monti – Milan (Italy)

Cluster headache is a serious problem, not least because its onset is often associated not so much with stress, as with relaxation. Let me get this straight.

If you have to take an exam, deliver a lecture, or perform any other activity that increases your stress and/or tension, in most cases the attack does not appear right away, but rather as soon as you relax.

If you are going through a time of great tension at work, then you go on vacation and suddenly relax (sleep longer and reduce tension quickly), cluster headache often strikes with more strength. This is why being unaware of this phenomenon puts CH sufferers in trouble (particularly in the early years of cluster headache suffering) and makes them suffer more, because it prevents them first from addressing the problem, i.e. the gradual relaxation phase, and then from resting and relaxing during breaks/holidays. All this triggers a vicious circle resulting from the generated distress that stimulates the activity of the hypothalamus, thus fostering the disease.

Today, our little Italian world is changing and somehow, alas, for the worse. We Italians have always considered research as the tail-light of the scientific community (for political reasons). The funds allocated to research have always been poor. Now, with the current economic crisis, the funds at stake are shrinking and, therefore, research on cluster headache is virtually non-existent.

Translated by Laura Monti – Milan (Italy)

The scientific community is thus at a standstill with respect to our illness.

Just think that CH sufferers realized, through the different OUCH branches founded in different countries around the world (OUCH USA, OUCH UK, OUCH Italy, OUCH Germany, etc.), that molecules of hallucinogenic drugs, such as psilocybe, LSD, and LSA, can be effective for the treatment of cluster headache and, in fact, in regions like America (more specifically Canada), the scientific community is also involved in the study of these new therapeutic approaches (see the relevant chapters).

On the other hand, unfortunately, nothing is said or done in Italy in this respect. One is even afraid to talk about them, because they are addictive drugs. Therefore no research is carried out at all. Please note that the effective doses are much lower than the "recreational" ones!

Far from me to try to encourage people to use them. I am simply providing an overview of the current situation, communicating a fact; in short, I am just trying to inform! Then every adult has his or her own choices to make, at his or her own risk, considering that the scientific community does not provide any support in this field, being illegal.

Translated by Laura Monti – Milan (Italy)

For more information about these drugs, their functioning, the effective molecules and dosages, please visit www.Clusterbuster.com, a spin-off of OUCH USA.

There is just one more thing I wish to tell on this subject. If you are new to cluster headache and have never submitted to conventional therapies, I recommend that you do not even consider using these psychotropic molecules. First rely on conventional drugs. CH sufferers that used these substances did so out of dissatisfaction with conventional therapies. If you consider using these substances, you should assess the possible subsequent psychiatric risk by reviewing your personal and family history of psychiatric disorders in order to minimize the risk of bringing them to the surface. If, and only if, you are drug-resistant and your life is unbearable because of CH, then you will decide whether it is really worth the risk.

In other countries, such as Germany, severe CH sufferers are prescribed doses of THC (tetrahydrocannabinol) as pills, with the purpose to mitigate the severity of the attacks and reduce the intake of Imigran® (see the chapter on THC).

While THC is known to be effective for many illnesses and for pain treatment, there are no advances in Italy in this respect. It is, at best, administered to terminally ill patients and, in recent years, it was prescribed for certain forms of multiple sclerosis.

This is unfortunately the poor state of research in Italy on the therapeutic use of certain types of drugs. We keep looking forward to future progress!

However, the world is changing, sometimes for the better, and today's widespread use of the internet helps you get out of isolation: you can interact with other CH sufferers in the forum, you can access information that was previously unavailable through a variety social networks (such as Facebook, YouTube, etc.), you can communicate with other CH sufferers located on the other side of the earth, where perhaps something new has been discovered. In short, you have many more opportunities of self-help than those available twenty years ago to CH sufferers!

This is the new reality of the twenty-first century; this is the positive aspect to be leveraged upon; this is the new way to go, still with a due critical approach and solely relying on information that comes from **competent and authoritative sources,** since the internet also contains unreliable information.

For this reason, it is important to be able to select information capable to promote our well-being; it is important to evaluate the *authoritativeness* of the source in order to receive valuable information.

Just consider the difference between the past and the present! Twenty years ago CH sufferers were alone, confined within their

Translated by Laura Monti – Milan (Italy)

own world. In the vast majority of cases they had no way to confront with others, because their illness was not as widespread as it is now (although its prevalence is increasing, particularly among women, something I predicted and posted many years ago in the OUCH forum).

I remember very well that, before meeting the four friends and co-founders of OUCH Italy (Riccardo Pentenero, Piera Ravazzoli, Stefano Capurro, and Valter Trovò) and, first and foremost, Riccardo, I would have paid any sum to meet another cluster sufferer like me to confront on everything I was going through, because crises are not just made of pain, but also generate neurovegetative problems, strange reactions in sexual activity, strange reactions to heat and cold, an amount of anger that is hard to manage, isolation, depression, etc.

I wanted to know what was happening to me, understand all the troubles I was going through. I wanted to confront and find logical links.

This is possible now, there is an opportunity to deal with the disease in the best possible way!

I started to pursue such opportunity more than ten years ago, and enjoy extraordinary benefits today. I will give you an idea, I will briefly tell you my story, and you can learn more by reading the book.

Translated by Laura Monti – Milan (Italy)

When CH first appeared, I had attacks. They were not too ravaging, all in all they were bearable, and persisted for some time between fifteen minutes to half an hour, however several times a day. At first I did not pay much attention and just thought to myself, "I must be tired." In fact my life was very stressful at the time, because of work.

Then the problem became more serious, pain was no longer bearable and, when it started, I had to stop anything I was doing. At first I manage the problem by myself with painkillers, but realized over time that they didn't work, that when pain subsided it was because the attack was over, not because of the painkillers. These recurring attacks during the day had a limited duration of about sixty to ninety minutes.

For quite some time – I still don't know why – I kept the whole thing to myself, as if it were something to be ashamed of! It then started to develop into something unbearable, something I could not hide, something that came and ravaged me, and at that point I began to seek medical help. I tried lots of physicians and got a not-too-accurate diagnosis. I took medications, sometimes useless for my disease, until one day a neurologist, who had a private practice in San Donato Milanese, made a more correct diagnosis!

Translated by Laura Monti – Milan (Italy)

He then introduced me to Imigran® and I was overjoyed, because I had finally found something that could help me get through that terrible pain.

I spent a lot of money, up to several millions of the old liras a year, to buy Imigran®. This was because 50% of its cost was charged to the patient until Rosi Bindi, the then Minister of Health, moved the medication to a different class.

In my attempt to understand this unreasonable pain, I approached other physicians, including a psychologist and an otolaryngologist. The latter submitted me to nose surgery for turbinate and septum reconstruction, also smoothing a small bone that interfered with the sphenopalatine ganglion in order to exclude any ear or nose involvement. Surgery brought significant benefits, however just in terms of breathing, not of headache!

In the process towards complete exclusion of nose or hear involvement, I tried with codeine and anesthetic applications on the sphenopalatine ganglion through the nasal pathway – something definitely unpleasant.

I tried homeopathy, iridology, pranotherapy, until I went to a "witchdoctor" and brought him my undershirt. In short, I was looking for any way, **I was desperate**, I could no longer live

Translated by Laura Monti – Milan (Italy)

because the disease was getting immensely worse and was by then chronic.

I tried to have it treated by a neurologist in Zingonia, Bergamo, specializing in headaches, including cluster headache, but my form became chronic and drug-resistant so that even all the lithium, verapamil, antiepileptic drugs, methysergide, and cortisone I took were no longer able to make my attacks subside. I then tried with cocktails of medications, but with no success.

At some point in 1998, I had a carotid echo doppler (at the Mondino headache center in Pavia) to assess the blood flow to the brain, which unveiled a thyroid cancer, a medullary cancer. So I went to the "Niguarda" hospital in Milan for total thyroidectomy, subtotal para-thyroidectomy, and laterocervical dissection: the attacks magically disappeared for some time (I did not understand why at that time, but now I do!).

The absence of attacks only persisted for some time, then it all started over again.

I met Riccardo, Sten, Piera, and Valter. That meeting aroused very strong emotions and CH magically disappeared for one week (keep these steps in mind, because they contain one of the keys to CH).

We founded the association together, and then organized the first OUCH Italy meeting with all the CH sufferers gathered

Translated by Laura Monti – Milan (Italy)

online. The meeting was marked by the enormous excitement about being solely with CH sufferers, and CH vanished for three days!

We then organized a trip to Vancouver, Canada, to attend the OUCH USA meeting. I brought my stock of Imigran®, but once again that strong emotion kept CH away.

At that time early trials were under way in America on the use of psilocybe and LSD, and I wanted to meet those researchers to make sure they were not mere quacks exploiting the issue. I actually met sensible people, well-dressed and well-bred family fathers – anything but quacks!

Back in Italy, CH returned as strong and violent as before, and over the years I was repeatedly hospitalized to try and tame the "beast".

Upon one of those day-hospital stays, a neurologist gave me trinitrin (a drug that generates fast and strong vasodilation) to make sure it was CH, and this caused a terrible attack that he was hardly able to control with oxygen or ergotamine injections. The next day, at home, I suffered a devastating attack that seemed to last forever, probably because of the prior intake of trinitrin. After ailing for seven hours, I took a double-barrel shotgun I had at home, loaded it with one cartridge, put it in my mouth, and shot. Click.

Translated by Laura Monti – Milan (Italy)

It all went black for a moment, then I realized I was still alive – and the attack had suddenly vanished! I had pulled the wrong trigger, the one operating the unloaded barrel! I suffered a strong emotional shock that made the attack subside instantly!

It was a very hard time for me, I could no longer live an ordinary life, I developed chronic anxiety and reactive depression. I could no longer sleep through the night because the attacks woke me up at all times. They also tended to appear when I woke up, so that I had to start the day with a shot of Imigran® to drag along in my everyday life.

Over the years I developed anger towards the world to a devastating and never-subsiding extent. The only way out I could see was suicide!

Meanwhile, through the association's activity, I came in touch with the scientific community and with highly skilled neurologists operating in top headache centers. One of them in particular – doctor Fabio Frediani – struck me for his great humanity, and I soon decided he should become my trusted neurologist (he still is).

I share everything with him, including my individual work with other CH sufferers, in the attempt to explain to him the common traits I believe I have identified and discovered. While he thought some of these were mere consequences of CH, others became

Translated by Laura Monti – Milan (Italy)

strategically important for the study of, and a new approach to the disease. **One, in particular, was the role of shocks and strong emotions, in both a positive and in a negative sense.**

We then decided to try a new method on me, which provided for causing me a shock.

We started with a direct drug-based shock (a bolus of cortisone at the hospital). It was indeed effective, but only for a short time.

We then tried reverse drug-based shock and, after some initial devastating exacerbation, CH magically surrendered, and disappeared after 26 days.

I then went through some tough events and experienced other very violent shocks (which I will detail later on in this book). I also did cause myself some other shocks deliberately, and these interacted with my CH and kept it away for some years.

After about 4 years, CH reappeared, both on the right and on the left side (whereas it only used to affect the right side before a strong traumatic event), responded to medications, and I just needed to take my effective dose of verapamil to stop an attack (intake occurred in a special way that no neurologist recommends, and that I will discuss further on in the book).

Translated by Laura Monti – Milan (Italy)

I often discussed with other people I am in contact with about knowing the disease and how to deal with it, who are better off than before. They haven't recovered, but they feel better, they suffer less, and their quality of life has improved. In some cases, this is because they used different medications or at different doses; in others because they were treated by highly skilled neurologists; in others yet, because they have become aware of and accepted the disease, and have "experienced" and addressed it with stronger and more effective weapons, or because they have learned new approaches, also drug-free, to "wear down" the disease and thus keep it more at bay and reduce suffering.

The message I intend to convey here is more simple than you might think: "By developing the right knowledge and following the right course, YOU CAN IMPROVE YOUR CONDITIONS, IF YOU WANT".

Just as I did, other people did too. YOU CAN MAKE IT! You too can get out of your loneliness. You too can live a better life and reduce your suffering. You too can make sure that this disease is no longer a substantial part of your life, but only a "bump in the road" and a minor element of your life.

What can you learn by reading this book with due attention and critical sense?

Translated by Laura Monti – Milan (Italy)

You can improve your knowledge of your disease, develop competence and know how, as well as the ability to confront with your neurologist to discuss it together, rather than just experience your relation as a passive one, because YOU are the best doctor for yourself! A mutual exchange with your neurologist is more effective.

You will get more information on treating centers. You will hear about methods other than allopathic medicine to struggle against your cluster headache. You will discover new ways to "wear down" the disease, because CH is a disease that affects you entirely – from your neurological system to your feelings, from your emotions to your thoughts... This often triggers vicious cycles that foster the disease. With knowledge, you will therefore enjoy the opportunity to act by stopping these vicious cycles.

Here is what you'll learn in a nutshell: you will learn that **you too can make it, if you want,** and if you make it, **I will be happy about having achieved my goal,** because I love you just because you suffer from CH, even if I never met you. I know what you're going through!

Aren't you a cluster headache sufferer, but rather a friend, a relative, a co-worker of a sufferer?

Translated by Laura Monti – Milan (Italy)

My book will offer valuable help to you too. It gives you the opportunity to get to learn about this disease, to understand sufferers, to learn the do's and don'ts to help and support them! A specific chapter is dedicated to you!

You are not a sufferer, nor a friend, a relative, or a co-worker, but a physician or medical scholar?

My book can help you grow in your profession. You will learn straight from a CH sufferer something that neurology schools may not have had the opportunity to teach you. You will also learn about the disease from points of view other than those you were taught, and you will improve your ability to abide by the oath you took – the "Hippocratic Oath" – by providing more effective help through the exercise of your profession.

Translated by Laura Monti – Milan (Italy)

CHAPTER I - IF YOU WANT, YOU CAN

The approach to **cluster headache** is going through a transitional phase in Italy. It is no longer like thirty years ago, when sufferers were seen as a rare breed, when you felt you were the only one affected and wondered in despair: "Why me?".

You would have paid gold to meet another cluster patient to share your suffering, to finally know someone that would understand you. Sadly, at that time the scientific community was close to helpless with respect to CH.

Today, however, and luckily, you are no longer alone; if you want, you can meet and talk to other CH sufferers. Today you have multiple forums to interact with fellow-sufferers (www.grappolaiuto.it and the www.cefalea.it forum), you can talk live on Facebook, you can watch explanatory videos on YouTube, etc.

The scientific community itself provides a variety of information websites. In short, today you can no longer say you are alone and don't know what to do and what you are suffering from. You can even self-diagnose your disease, because the CH diagnosis is actually easier than you may think, being strictly based on your symptoms.

Translated by Laura Monti – Milan (Italy)

Talking about self-diagnosis, I recently read about a guy that self-diagnosed his CH by reading the OUCH Italy forum and confronting with other participants in the forum.

Certain concepts in the book are restated and repeated several times to ensure they are perfectly understood, and this concept I am conveying (the isolation connected with the "why me" thought, I have no one to share it with and be understood) is not an ordinary one, because it concerns the removal of a factor that used to trigger a vicious cycle feeding CH.

Things have changed also because of the advent of technology. Communication and information systems were multiplied exponentially with the introduction and growing popularity of the internet.

Today it is easier than ever before to communicate in real time from one part of the world to the other. It is easier than ever before to collect sensitive information (such as the information available online) on the use of hallucinogenic drugs for the treatment of CH. If you wish, you can know in real time when the next meetings of OUCH USA or the information conventions of Clusterbuster will take place, or better still, the meetings of OUCH Italy, much easier to access.

However, we are still far from a real turning point, still going through a transitional phase where, finally, in most headache

Translated by Laura Monti – Milan (Italy)

centers, "CH" is acknowledged and we know which are the right medications to treat it. However, for example, some centers still don't know how to use oxygen to deal with the symptoms or, if they do know, use low doses, which (sadly) are not effective for CH, and thus only give partial help.

We are going through a transitional phase because today some (general) practitioners are still not fully informed about this illness and its context, with subsequent diagnosis-related issues.

Note that YOU make the difference in this transition. Your attitude and behavior can make a difference! *Is it clear?*

The bad news, in this chapter, is that if you isolate yourself, if you surrender to depression, if you don't interact with others, if you don't use the information channels that are easily accessible through the internet, if you don't take direct action proactively ... you can only fall back two decades, when things were definitely worse, patients suffered more, and received no support, including psychological.

Another bad piece of news for you is that brain biochemistry changes and neuroendocrine system rebalancing are slow processes. So, if you expect to get positive results as soon as you start this transformation, you will be disappointed and will tend to discontinue this new course. If you make that mistake, you will be a loser! **You must be aware of this and hold on!**

Translated by Laura Monti – Milan (Italy)

If you want your CH to improve by simply making a first attempt at changing medications, trying to use meditation for a week (the usefulness of which is discussed further on in the book), or starting to change a bad habit, but without persisting, you will hardly succeed.

You have to read the book, absorb it, try over and over again. You have to keep reading the proposed solutions and try them over and over again, because what may not have worked a couple of years ago may work now.

Throughout our life we keep evolving and changing; therefore, the same medications you developed tolerance for, if not taken for some time, can become effective again. **Please, don't forget it!**

A new approach adapted to the situation is now necessary, useful, and effective. **You have to take control of your life; you have to take control of your CH; you have to deal with physicians in a more knowledgeable and effective way.**

When dealing with them you should take an active attitude, rather than passive and submissive. Today you should also use the non-medical techniques that I am going to reveal further on in the book, which offer practical help to change the course of your CH and are part of what I call "**wearing down**".

Translated by Laura Monti – Milan (Italy)

Today, IF YOU WANT, YOU CAN, but you have to want. You have to take action, you have to participate in the existing forums, you have to develop a culture of your own disease, **YOU HAVE TO ACCEPT THAT YOU SUFFER FROM CH** (capitalized, because this is the first step most people do not manage to take). Let me repeat this, <u>**you have to accept your CH,**</u> you should not reject or fight it neurotically, you should not be ashamed of it. It is like any other illness, and others will understand if they want to, otherwise who cares!

What I invite you to do in this chapter is to take an *active* and *positive* attitude towards your illness, to become a major player, to **take control by following a course of transformation and change that will benefit you forever.**

I now invite you to dwell on a concept that will be useful in your life, not just for your CH: if you want to change your life, change three habits a year – just three – and you will see that the course of your life will take a new turn. Replace three negative habits with three positive ones (so that you will not feel a sense of void).

Write them down at home and at work so that you can see and read them several times a day, lest you forget, so that they help strengthen your willingness to act, because over time you will be highly motivated on some days and less in others. In this latter case, you will tend to forget about your good intentions and fall back into the three bad habits that you are trying to change. This exercise should be repeated for at least twenty-eight days (two months would be even better), which is the time required to consolidate the new "synapses" (the functional connections between two nerve cells or between a nerve cell and the peripheral organ of reaction) through which the paths of new habits run. By doing so, they will be rooted in your memory, unconsciously!

I say these things to you and invite you to take this attitude in order to continue the journey on a new path, because this is what I did, and it worked. Because this is what some other CH sufferers did with me, and it worked.

It took me years to understand these things. No one had paved the way for me before, I had to pave my own. It was a very hard job, though: checks and counterchecks to ensure that things would work; mistakes, falls, slips were constantly with me along the way. This is why it took me so long.

What I am trying to do for you with this book is to show you the paved way, so that you can follow it and know what is most effective and lasting for you.

Translated by Laura Monti – Milan (Italy)

Just think that it took me a long time (about five years) to realize that shocks were effective. Early remissions happened by chance after very strong but positive emotional events, and then events that caused strong negative shocks occurred. I also tried direct drug-based shock and then the reverse shock. Based on my early certainties, I sought confirmation by taking the shock-based approach using psilocybe. It happened again following a very serious motorcycle accident (obviously unwanted), where I suffered a strong brain concussion and three brain hemorrhages. I no longer recognized people, I had eight broken vertebrae and had my arm reconstructed. Then came a shock due to very serious surgery I had to undergo for a second esophageal cancer (my esophagus was removed alongside the relevant vagus nerve branches, the stomach was taken out, cut out, reconstructed with a tube-shape; two arteries out of three were eliminated, and the stomach was directly connected with my throat). In this case, too, the event was unwanted, but the shock I suffered was very strong, starting with simple general anesthesia for one day of surgery, followed by five days of resuscitation and a variety of post-surgery complications. On all these occasions, my CH went into remission for variable periods of time. By then it had actually been chronic for many years and, when it reappeared, it was still chronic!

Translated by Laura Monti – Milan (Italy)

In short, before telling you that shocks interact with CH, I assure you that I have first analyzed and experienced this in person. At the same time, I sought the same confirmation through an interaction with other CH sufferers, who participated in the individual meetings I described in the introduction, and they confirmed too: *"Yes, I too had a remission when my father died,"* *"Yes, I too had a remission when I broke up with my wife,"* *"Yes, I too had a remission after I suffered a scary accident,"* *"Yes, I had CH and it magically vanished after I was hospitalized."*

It should be noted that shocks, particularly if emotional, arouse strictly subjective reactions. A family bereavement can be a shock for some, but not for others. Moving to a new house can be a shock for some, but not for others. There are dozens of similar examples to explain how subjectively an event can be considered as shocking.

Translated by Laura Monti – Milan (Italy)

CHAPTER II - MY STORY OF CHALLENGES AND SUCCESSES

WHY THIS CHAPTER?

In this chapter I will tell you my story from the beginning, from the time I was first visited by the beast to the time it became a devastating tragedy, which ruined my existence until I managed to tame it.

I will try to bring back all the memories to my mind, but I probably will not be able to follow the right timeline because my mind is no longer as clear as it used to be. The damage I suffered from three brain hemorrhages, and maybe also from headache, in addition to ageing, has significantly weakened my memory skills. Nevertheless the strongest memories are carved in my history, and therefore I will tell you about them as accurately as possible. I want to try to make you understand what I have been through, my story of difficulties, my story of how I found solutions and achieved successes I can savor today because they have radically changed the quality of my life!

CH is an extremely subjective illness, in that it affects each person's life in extremely personal domains. CH is an all-encompassing disease, it is influenced by neurology, brain biochemistry, thoughts, and emotions and, since each of us is unique, this subjectivity is just natural.

Translated by Laura Monti – Milan (Italy)

CH is not like diabetes, which is easily controlled with adequate doses of insulin. CH is a disease that must be controlled by acting on different spheres, including medicine, quality of life, sleep-wake cycles, stress, sports, meditation, thinking and, last but not least, emotions, which you should also manage to control.

This is to explain that **I don't expect that what was good for me is also good for you**. This is absolutely not the case. But my "wear down" experience, which needs to be customized for you, is anyway a weapon at your disposal, and you should use it.

I want you to understand that you cannot just rely on your doctor or on medications to counter this disease, but relying on yourself, taking control of your life, painstakingly and constantly using all the available weapons to tame the beast is much more effective. By doing so, you can also achieve enormous improvements with respect to your CH, as well as a transformation that you can hardly imagine now, if you are desperately suffering for your attacks. You have to restore your hope and trust, accept your disease, live with it, and confine it to the mere time of the attack, rather than experience it as if it were always there, constantly in your thoughts.

You have to find your way to restore maximum balance with respect to life and you will see that all this acting, rather than surrendering (such as taking medicines or relying entirely on your neurologist), will strike and gradually weaken your beast.

Translated by Laura Monti – Milan (Italy)

Mind that in some cases the beast is a sign of a lack of balance, but such balance can be restored, because it is an intrinsic tendency of nature itself.

I wish to dedicate this chapter to you in order to let you get an insight of my suffering, to share with you all my sensitive data in view of encouraging you by arousing your awareness of the fact that there are so many people that suffer, but **the attitude we take towards suffering and health issues can make a clear difference – the very difference that can make you win.**

HOW MY ORDEAL BEGAN - "EPISODIC CLUSTER HEADACHE WITHOUT A PROPER DIAGNOSIS"

When my beast first visited me, it was a tame, sneaky beast, which gave no sign of its atrocity and its dangerousness. I had pain in the head that always began from the corner between the brow ridge and the nasal root, beyond the inside corner of the eye – always on the right, never on the left.

This pain subsided if I pressed that point, the trigger that starts the pain. It lasted for a short time, about fifteen to twenty minutes, and was quite bearable, to the extent that it did not prevent my continuing to do what I was doing. It was painful, of course, but endurable.

Translated by Laura Monti – Milan (Italy)

I noticed right away that these micro-attacks occurred at fixed times, but did not give too much importance to this at first, and mostly attributed the reason for this pain to tiredness.

Time went by and pain recurred, roughly at the same times of the day, except that its duration increased to thirty/forty minutes and up to an hour.

I started to feel annoyed, sometimes the pain was hardly bearable, and that was when I first went for medications. At first I took ordinary painkillers and saw that pain subsided – after an hour, on average.

At some point in time, it vanished completely, and I stopped thinking about it.

After a few months it returned. Again, the pain started quite mildly, then got stronger day after day, and its duration gradually increased. I continued to take ordinary painkillers, but realized – time and again – that pain did not subside even after one and a half or two yours, despite the medications. I soon realized that these medications were not effective and tried others, but still with the same result – no effect!

For some time I had such strange headaches I hardly managed to treat, which were causing me some trouble, because the pain was significant and did not allow me to continue devoting to my tasks.

Translated by Laura Monti – Milan (Italy)

That is how my **cluster headache** came about, an episodic cluster headache that appeared for about a month, or a month and a half, twice a year. Of course, at that time I was still unaware of what it was and had never seen a neurologist.

A few months later the problem recurred, at first with mild and bearable attacks, which gradually developed into more and more challenging and painful ones. I explained the situation to my GP and he promptly referred me to a neurologist.

The first neurologist I saw did not diagnose cluster headache immediately. He recognized it as a headache and gave me medications – I don't remember which – to counter it. When I saw the neurologist, the cluster was already subsiding and the attacks were characteristically less violent. Of course we thought it was the effect of the medications I was taking, and he advised me to continue with those medications over time.

At some point in time I noticed I was suffering no more attacks and discontinued drug intake. Time went by, and the pain reappeared, much more aggressive.

I coped with the umpteenth cluster arguing with the neurologist, who claimed I had made a mistake by discontinuing drug intake; he therefore prescribed the same medications again and invited me not to discontinue their intake even if the attacks vanished.

Translated by Laura Monti – Milan (Italy)

This continued through a few clusters, with me not always closely complying with the prescription, until the need was such that I had to become compliant and careful to the extent that I could demonstrate that those medications were of no use and that, on average, at season changes, I suffered this pain that no medication seemed to be able to stop.

If we focus for a moment on the times of the year when my cluster headache attacks appeared, namely at season changes, we can clearly see that at those times the body undergoes environmental stress, to which the hypothalamus must react with physical adaptation to the environmental change.

One day, while I was being examined by my doctor, I happened to suffer an attack. He gave me a subcutaneous injection of anesthetic (in the scalp) and the pain soon subsided. Who knows whether it was for the injection or it would have vanished anyway!

This doctor was a private physician, who was so powerless and disappointed for not being able to help me that he decided to charge me nothing for his examinations. Thank-you, Doc!

Each time I tried to pay for his examination, he said: "Davide, when you become a wealthy entrepreneur you will pay." The examinations got more and more frequent, because the problem was becoming very serious. Twice a year I was really sick for

Translated by Laura Monti – Milan (Italy)

some time, not yet from the devastating attacks I would suffer later, but because the pain tended to become unbearable!

I mentioned the free examinations because we CH sufferers are often full of anger for our suffering, and sometimes get mad at doctors and pour out this anger on them for being unable to heal us. However we should admit that most of them do so in good faith; they would like to help us but fail, and we get mad at them in return (albeit understandably).

This doctor was not able to help me with the right diagnosis, but I will always remember him for his humanity and devotion and am still grateful to him!

Cluster headache attacks continued to come twice a year, each time more excruciating, and that is when the ordeal really began!

They came when I was on holiday, which they spoilt. They came when I was out with friends and forced me to go home, thus spoiling my evening. They came every time I enjoyed a beer (but I was still unaware of the link between alcohol intake and the attacks). They came at times of intimacy with my partner, stopping me and overwhelming me with pain and suffering. The attacks began to show their atrocity and I soon felt helpless and frightened!

Translated by Laura Monti – Milan (Italy)

This generated anger – anger for not understanding why I was suffering, anger for suffering, anger as a reaction to this suffering; an anger that soon turned against my very life, which had become almost impossible to live!

At that time I was suffering from sinusitis, so I thought, couldn't the cause of these attacks be an otolaryngological disorder?

I saw an outstanding otolaryngologist, who promptly observed I had breathing troubles – frontal and right maxillary sinusitis. He prescribed investigations and discovered a right-side maxillary polyp, as well as a deviated nasal septum. He thought the cause of my migraine could have a rhinogenic origin and suggested surgery.

I had surgery, he straightened my nasal septum, fixed my turbinates, cleaned out my sinusitis, and smoothed a bone that, in his opinion, interfered with the sphenopalatine ganglion. Expectations were good and headache, if actually due to sinusitis, should then disappear.

Disappear my foot! The beast regularly returned at season changes and made me suffer more and more!

I started to feel out of sorts and to have negative thoughts, with a tendency to depression. "Why me?" I used to repeat to myself... "What wrong did I do to deserve this ordeal? What is it

Translated by Laura Monti – Milan (Italy)

that is happening to me? Help! I'm scared! I'm scared! I can't live through this!"

At that time I lived with my father, who was incredulous, grieved, and terrified by this situation. He had already lost a son, who had woken up one night shouting "Ow... my head!" and then had fainted without ever recovering. It was back in 1967 and he was thought to have suffered from an acute viral encephalitis. That poor man was then looking at his younger son writhing in pain from headache, bumping his head into the wall, cursing like mad, and exploding in devastating rage during the most acute attacks. What a terrible suffering it must have been for him, too!

Dad suffered with me, but he did so silently; he knew that, when I was locked up in my room with an attack, he should leave me alone, he should not even ask me, *How are you? How's it going? Did you get over it?* "No no, leave me alone," I used to answer, "leave me alone!". I lived in my pain, in my suffering, and could share it with no one.

I don't know why, but I didn't talk about it to anyone then, I hid it, as if I were to blame!

When it subsided, I went back to him with a harrowed, sometimes swollen face, I had serum rashes on my right upper eyelid that swelled my eye as if stung by a wasp. Meanwhile I stuffed myself with suppositories that the neurologist prescribed against pain, but that in fact were not effective.

At that time I had learned to counter CH with my own methods. First of all I had identified some triggers, i.e. points on the head that, if pressed with my fingers, produced some benefit – indeed very mild, but something positive, at least. It is a shame that sometimes, when searching for these triggers on my head, I found points that, if pressed, made the pain even worse. However, the most effective points included one at the usual point of origin of pain, i.e. at the intersection between the nose and the brow ridge, in the inner region above the corner of the eye.

Another useful point was behind the ear and on the small bunch behind the nape of the neck; there are two of these bunches, one on the right and one on the left and, of course, I pressed the one on the right because my attacks were always on the right. I later found out that these are acupuncture and shiatsu acupressure triggers.

During the most violent attacks, I also learned to sit on the bed in a strange position, i.e. I would bend my head with my chin close to my neck and sit on my knees with my butt upwards, loading weight onto my head and forcing it to bend towards my chin and my sternum. While doing so I listened to the pain with the utmost attention, virtually starting meditation in pain and

Translated by Laura Monti – Milan (Italy)

becoming one thing with it. When I succeeded, I entered into a state of trance in which suffering vanished, although the pain was still there. This only happened a few times, but many others I didn't succeed, I was pissed off and bumped my fists and my head in the walls and cabinets.

However, even when this approach succeeded, a doorbell or an intercom ringing, or Dad entering the room to see how I was doing (in fact, he learned not to do it again) were enough to take me out of that state of trance and bring back the pain as strong as ever. I learnt to do this spontaneously and randomly, and only later found out it is actually meditation in pain.

When I returned to the otolaryngologist for a check, I received a proposal to exclude any rhinogenic cause: he suggested that I submit to a treatment that provided for introducing a flexible metal device into my nose with a dose of anesthetic and cocaine on the tip, to be applied to the sphenopalatine ganglion. *The goal was to partially put the ganglion to sleep. If the pain had an ophthalmic origin, it would subside!*

I was convinced, and went to submit to these applications while having a cluster headache. You can just imagine how disturbing it was, though not at all if compared with the pain I felt. Therefore I endured the nuisance and continued with the applications! No result. After an adequate number of applications, the doctor

Translated by Laura Monti – Milan (Italy)

himself told me to stop, having excluded any involvement within his scope.

This second hope of healing was lost too, and my mood was at the lowest. I was enraged and started to become seriously depressed!

A FEW YEARS LATER, THERE COMES THE CLUSTER HEADACHE DIAGNOSIS.

One day, while I was in hospital for other reasons, I suffered a violent attack. A neurologist was summoned, examined me, and suggested for the first time it was cluster headache.

I left the hospital and started treatment with him – he owned a headache center. The first time I went to his headache center I was asked countless questions and had to fill countless questionnaires, and was **then diagnosed with episodic cluster headache.**

The professor immediately gave me Carbolithium®, a lithium-salt based medication prescribed for manic depressive psychosis, bipolar depression, and as a mood stabilizer. I started taking this medication and checking my lithium blood levels to prevent the risk of intoxication.

The medication had a somewhat mitigating effect, but did not help me get over my headache and left me with a number of

Translated by Laura Monti – Milan (Italy)

disturbing side effects – by then my emotional sphere was flat and nothing perturbed me; however I got used to them and continued with this medication for years, trying to partially make up for these troubles.

At that time, I worked at a construction site in Calabria – southern Italy – and started to experience strange neurovegetative disorders: my body thermoregulation system had failed. I remember waking up in full summer with a freezing cold feeling that persisted for the first half hour; then, during an attack, I felt damned hot and transpired abundantly, and then I went back to feeling cold when the attack subsided.

Because I was in charge of safety at the construction site, during the day I kept driving along the natural gas pipeline track in an off-road vehicle, and while driving I often suffered severe and overwhelming narcolepsy-like sleep surges. In that case I had to stop, and fell asleep in a flash. I woke up a few minutes later, five, maybe ten. That was quite strange, as well as dangerous, considering that the Salerno-Reggio Calabria highway had no emergency lane!

Despite being crushed by pain and fatigue, after a violent attack I experienced very intense and long-lasting erections and wondered, *"What the hell is happening to me? Why are all these things happening to me? Is it because of the headache? What if I had brain cancer?"*.

Translated by Laura Monti – Milan (Italy)

In short, I was no longer at peace. I was a real cluster headache sufferer. I had an early onset of neurasthenia and fear never left me – the fear of another attack!

I kept thinking about it obsessively, thus triggering a vicious cycle of negative thinking, negative emotion, anger, and fear about the future – all emotional components that, as I later learned, feed the beast.

It was torture, it was like living in a nightmare, and the clusters were starting to last longer and longer.

Pain was too much, and its frequency too. During an attack, I changed completely, I turned into a desperate, depressed person, and began to see death as a liberation from this evil. The thought of suicide was my way out and I kept saying to myself, *"Davide, when you can't take it anymore, kill yourself and get over with it."* This thought was more and more frequent during the attacks, it was the only way out I could think of, but then, when the attack subsided and I got hold of myself again, I would say, *"What the hell are you thinking? Are you mad?"* In short, two opposite visions of life while having and not having an attack. Over time and following studies on psychology that I made to further develop my culture, I understood **the reason for such terrible thoughts**: the thought of suicide was a "sort of psychological inherent self-help" that gave me the strength to cope with the day and live in the present from day to day. Living with the thought of such a life of suffering for many years ahead would have been psychologically unsustainable. This approach is, in fact, adopted in drug rehab centers, where patients are taught to resist temptation for one day at a time. Addiction to drugs, video games, people (addictive love), social networks, etc. has nothing to do with cluster headache, but the strategy I adopted was aimed at the same psychological aspect of coping with a tough thought and expectation challenge, which would generate a loser's emotions.

The attacks were ravaging, they transformed me completely!

Over time I was also prescribed cortisone vials, which were effective at countering the attacks but, unfortunately, could not stop the cluster, so that when I started to scale it down towards withdrawal, the attacks reappeared. There were periods in time when I had cortisone shots to enjoy some respite from this dreadful disease.

THE DISTANCE BETWEEN SAYING AND DOING IS HUGE, AND DESPAIR MAKES YOU CROSS IT WITH A "LITTLE JUMP" – I DECIDE TO GO FOR SUICIDE

One day, during an outpatient visit at a hospital, I was given trinitrin, a strong vasodilator used in cardiology, as well as to confirm the cluster headache diagnosis. Shortly after the intake I

Translated by Laura Monti – Milan (Italy)

suffered a devastating attack that did not subside. I had a shot of dihydroergotamine (a vasoconstrictor), but the attack persisted. I was administered oxygen for several minutes, but the attack persisted. After about three and a half hours, it vanished, and I went home, a ravaged man, to sleep.

The next day I had another devastating and persistent attack at home, probably because of the intake of trinitrin the day before. After suffering for seven hours, I got hold of a dual-barrel shotgun I had at home, loaded it with one cartridge, stuck it into my mouth, and shot. Click. Everything went black for a moment, then I realized I was still alive and that the attack had suddenly vanished! I had pulled the wrong trigger and operated the unloaded barrel! I suffered a strong emotional shock. **At the moment I did not associate the occurrence with the shock I experienced,** I was stunned by what had happened, I felt exhausted and not very clear-headed, I put away my father's rifle and threw myself into bed to sleep. It was afternoon, and I slept through to the next day!

On the next day I could not believe what I had done and it remained my personal secret for years, but I started to be clear about something – **the strong emotion I had suffered in the instant I was sure I would die had stopped the attack as if by operating a switch - "on or off."** Something had happened then at an emotional level that had completely removed the attack,

Translated by Laura Monti – Milan (Italy)

an attack that had lasted for hours, something extraordinary because they usually lasted a maximum of two hours, sometimes with residual pain, albeit not of the same intensity as the actual attack.

MY EXPERIENCE IN THE HYPERBARIC CHAMBER

In the face of my conditions, operators at the headache center where I was being treated suggested that I use a hyperbaric chamber, which they had found to be effective in some cases of cluster headache.

They virtually assumed it was effective to spend about an hour and a half with a higher partial oxygen pressure in the blood.

I started the process. The hyperbaric chamber was in the neighborhood of Bergamo, but back then I lived in San Donato Milanese. From the logistic point of view, this meant I had to use an entire afternoon to reach the premises a few minutes before the scheduled time, register, enter the hyperbaric chamber, wait for pressurization to reach about 1.5 bar, breathe through a face mask for an hour and a half, then wait for chamber depressurization, exit, wait about twenty minutes before I could leave the center, pick up my car, and drive home. It meant using most of the afternoon. I may be wrong, but I think I went there

Translated by Laura Monti – Milan (Italy)

every day or every two days. It was a real nuisance, but I accepted this "important engagement" too if it could set me free from those devastating attacks.

I had multiple hyperbaric chamber sessions, but still had the attacks. I had enough, to hell the hyperbaric chamber! Anger surged, *but why is there nothing that works for me?*

TRY AGAIN, YOU'LL BE LUCKIER! TOUGH LUCK!

At that point I decided to take an entirely different approach. I knew the Chinese professor who had imported acupuncture in Italy. He had treated my mother before she passed away and had managed to help her. I decided to give a try to acupuncture!

I went to Via Vallazze, Milan, in the Lambrate neighborhood, and had their acupuncture check-up. I was found to have headache, anxiety, and depression. I started to submit to acupuncture sessions, very expensive in consideration of our economic conditions, and my headache increased dramatically. They claimed it was just natural and I had to be patient, but I couldn't. In consideration of the poor results and of the costs I was incurring I decided to stop. However over time I spoke with some CH sufferers that benefited from acupuncture, so maybe I was wrong to stop!

Translated by Laura Monti – Milan (Italy)

THE DISCOVERY OF SUMATRIPTAN

I finally discovered the existence of **sumatriptan succinate in vials**, or Imigran®. I tried it and noticed that the attacks subsided within a few minutes. However I suffered from severe (but very severe) side effects, particularly after the first doses. Such effects included neck, head, and shoulder strain, breathing difficulties, and exhaustion, but they were nothing compared to a CH attack, which then vanished within a few minutes.

Thus I became a regular Imigran® consumer and, despite having prophylactic therapies, I had an average of two to three shots a day.

Back then, the drug cost 118,000 liras[2] and was a class B drug, i.e. 50% of its price was charged to the patient. In economic terms, I was ruined.

When I worked at construction sites, mostly in the south of Italy, I always had troubles at getting the medication. I had to find a doctor on site to obtain a prescription, but most doctors did not even know what it was. I had to argue and quarrel until I found a

---

[2] One Euro = 1,936.27 liras

Translated by Laura Monti – Milan (Italy)

doctor who understood my case and gave me regular prescriptions. I kept going to the doctor's clinic looking for Imigran® and my arms had turned purple because of the countless shots I had. But **Imigran® was always effective for me and always stopped my attacks!**

I remember how many times, before joining construction site meetings or performing any tasks, I sensed an upcoming attack and had to have a shot, then gathered all my strength to continue with my job. I didn't give up, I did my best, I turned anger into strength, but the level of stress I suffered was definitely devastating and fostered my CH (though back then I was unaware).

I spent up to ten million liras a year to buy Imigran® and was in real trouble. My health conditions demanded that I keep away from the stress I was under at the construction site, but I couldn't because I needed the extra money I earned to buy Imigran® and, if I returned to Milan, my basic salary as an employee would not have been enough! By then "my beast had chronicized."

MY BOSS: STRESS

Stress levels were very high at work because, although I was exhausted from CH, I performed a job that on one hand I

Translated by Laura Monti – Milan (Italy)

enjoyed and gave me satisfaction, but on the other caused me enormous stress.

I worked every day, including on Saturdays and Sundays, for about twelve to fourteen hours a day and I often went out at night to follow the escorts of HGVs that carried sidebooms (pipe-laying tractors) and excavators (all illegal activities that the top management of the site forced me to carry out at my own risk).

On the other hand, during the day I supervised work along the gas pipeline. I dealt with public bodies (INAIL,[3] healthcare companies, hospitals, municipal, regional and provincial authorities). I provided training courses on safety to all our employees. I held safety meetings on all work stages. I dealt with clients and kept arguing with contractors and subcontractors to ensure their compliance with safety rules. At those location and at that time, safety at work was by all means neglected, particularly by contractors/subcontractors, and I had to keep "breathing down their back" and argue to get practical results and receive monthly safety records. I remember that sometimes I even blackmailed them and withheld their progress of work balance, which they needed to collect payment, until they delivered the required safety records. This was illegal, but I was forced to adopt unorthodox and conflicting strategies to achieve the positive result that was needed to protect the health of the

---

[3] The Italian national institute for insurance against industrial injuries.

Translated by Laura Monti – Milan (Italy)

workers and obtain statistical data to complete analyses and improvements. In Machiavelli's words, "the ends justify the means!"

One weekend I worked and the next I drove to Milan in my car to spend time with my girlfriend and Dad. Just twenty-four hours, then back to the south by car, for a total of two thousand kilometers in a weekend. My lifestyle did not match my physiological needs.

I was threatened, I was delivered a rabbit's entrails on my doormat, and my dog that I always took with me was hanged. He was a stray puppy, I had raised him with bottle feeding, and I adored him. A shower of punches would have hurt me less!

Nevertheless, I did not give up, I leveraged on the anger and aggressiveness I had developed within and managed to get what I wanted to ensure safety and thus protect those that worked hard to earn their living.

However this kind of life meant too much stress for me. I liked it, because I always turned out a winner and the site managers were satisfied with my work to the extent that they competed for me in multiple sites, until they managed to put me in charge of several sites at the same time. But I had been caught in a loop that fed my beast, because my lifestyle was definitely unbalanced and did not meet my physiological needs.

Translated by Laura Monti – Milan (Italy)

I DON'T GIVE UP AND TRY A DIFFERENT APPROACH.

I heard about the "Besta" hospital as an excellent headache center and decided to try and see if they could help me. I asked for an appointment via the national healthcare service, and got one after about eight months with a lady doctor whose name I am not going to mention for privacy reasons (not least because I have nothing positive to say about her).

She finally received me for a check that was absolutely outrageous – a five-minute chat to decide that my headache was not cluster headache and prescribe medications for vasomotor headache. She quickly dismissed me after giving me a phone number for use in case of need, and making a follow-up appointment after four months.

Meanwhile things did not improve, the prescribed medications were completely ineffective and I decided to contact her before the end of the four months. I tried several times but in vain, the service didn't work, there was no way to reach her. I was very disappointed about the national healthcare service. I got angry and decided to forget about her, stop taking the prescribed medications, and never see her again.

Translated by Laura Monti – Milan (Italy)

That said, the "Besta" is, indeed, an excellent headache center, as I found out later on when I met highly skilled and professional doctors. The problem was I had just fallen in the wrong hands.

BACK TO THE OLD TREATMENTS AND EARLY NON-MEDICINAL APPROACHES

I reverted to my darlings Carbolithium® and Imigran® - when needed, which meant daily because my case had developed into chronic drug-resistant cluster headache.

It was quite a quick transformation, probably fueled by my lifestyle **and the abuse of Imigran®.** In fact, a few years later, when OUCH Italy was founded, I began the personal work described in the introduction and started confronting with others in the forum. **We realized that, according to our opinion and experience, the abuse of Imigran® tends to result into the beast's chronicization.**

Of course this is not a certainty, but an observation that the association has made over time through mutual confrontation. Many people have observed a worsening of their CH connected with the intake of high doses of Imigran®. Several factors could be responsible for this: first, the characteristics of the medication, which has only limited historical data, being in use

Translated by Laura Monti – Milan (Italy)

for just one generation (Imigran® was launched in the 1990s); second, drug poisoning (the most reliable assumption according to the scientific community); third, the beast should be allowed to pour out its strength, if you stop it, it comes back stronger than before. It is a form of accumulated energy that needs to be discharged, a message that the "body's intelligence" should convey (the holistic vision).

Though being truly disappointed, I am not one that gives up. I heard about a kind of Chinese guru that treated people using oriental techniques. He had a center in Pesaro, in central Italy, so I arranged a visit to ask for his opinion. I travelled to Pesaro, slept there with other people, participated in the morning massage sessions, and then came question time. I raised my hand and was given the floor. I said I constantly suffered from headache and was no longer able to bear this agony. The guru asked me, "Are you having a headache now?" and I said, "No, I'm not having a headache now". He got angry in return, raised his voice, and shouted I had made an overstatement by saying I constantly suffered from headache. I should not say constantly because constantly means all day long.

The way he had answered aroused some sort of dislike in me, because he hadn't even let me explain what these attacks were like and that they came repeatedly every day. He told me the cause of these attacks was a load of energy that I could not

Translated by Laura Monti – Milan (Italy)

discharge and that I could recover by walking 25km a day barefoot! I thought he was mad and left without ever returning and speaking to him. He was definitely unpleasant: first he shouted at me, then told me I had to walk barefoot to counter the attacks. I couldn't believe it and thought, what a quack! But then I thought he could be right according to a holistic vision, though of course I never went walking 25 km barefoot every day because I didn't trust what he said, and moreover it was logistically impossible for me to do so, considering my lifestyle.

While working at the Montodine construction site near Cremona, I travelled every day back and forth. One morning I had a strong attack just before holding a training course for new hires. I went to hide in my makeshift office in a container, crouching between the cabinet and the wall to live through my attack, waiting for it to subside. However the attack got worse and the only way out was a vial of Imigran®. I could not afford to let it continue, because I was supposed to hold the training course.

Meanwhile a new hire, a guy in his fifties, entered my office and saw me lying on the floor in pain. I asked him to leave and he politely moved away and stood in front of the door to stop other new hires from entering, because the staff manager, based in another makeshift office, referred them to me.

The attack subsided, I washed my face, I used my strength and anger like fuel to move on and held the course as I was supposed

Translated by Laura Monti – Milan (Italy)

to do. At the end I felt I had to thank that man, who had seen I was sick and had stopped others from entering. I explained my case to him, he thought it over, and told me the story of his mother, who had been diagnosed with metastasized breast cancer with a life expectancy of few months. That woman had then turned to a Belgian iridologist, who also treated the Ukrainian army, allegedly with extraordinary results. He had treated and healed his mother from cancer and she still had both her breasts, which doctors had said should have been removed!

This gave me new hope. I wanted to try myself, but was discouraged by the language and the distance. That man spoke French and put me in contact with his sister, who worked in Belgium and had already been in contact with the iridologist for their mother.

I was asked to take a macro photo of my eyes and send it to him along with some vials with reagents I had to fill with my blood.

I was so desperate that one Saturday morning, after receiving the vials to fill, I squeezed my arm with my belt, made my vein swell, and took a blood sample by myself! I filled the vials and sent them with the photos to Ategis in Brussels.

After a while, I got a diagnosis: intestinal inflammation, infection, massive intoxication, leg circulation, kidneys, decalcification,

Translated by Laura Monti – Milan (Italy)

blood quality, right lung upper and middle lobe, liver and bile, low pressure, throat, and thyroid.

He wrote so many things that some were just right. Indeed I had kidney stones, my pressure has actually always been low, and I have bradycardia. In 1998 I had cancer, a thyroid medullary carcinoma. I'm not persuaded, I said to myself. I had turned to him for headache but he didn't even mention it in his diagnosis. Strange, but it was a new approach and I wanted to try it. Through that man's sister I was prescribed the treatment and ordered it for a fairly high amount of money.

The treatment was amazing! I received several vials containing liquids made up of elements of the periodic table, as well as tablets. The compounds should be taken on an empty stomach and it took more than two hours to complete the treatment, because those compounds should be taken by pouring them in a teaspoon, strictly made of plastics, a quarter of an hour apart. I had to be in Crema as early as at 6.45 a.m., so I got up early, but this treatment called for some heavy work. I started, continued for a while, got no benefits, and gave up. I admit I didn't manage to properly complete the treatment, but I had taken about three-quarters of the vials, so I was about to finish. I don't know whether I would have achieved any benefits if I had completed it, but the mere fact of having to wake up so early in the morning was a stress as such for me. I didn't get enough sleep. In short, it

Translated by Laura Monti – Milan (Italy)

didn't work, and I also abandoned iridology. Of course, I was surprised about him mentioning my thyroid and then having thyroid cancer in 1998.

PRANOTHERAPY AND THE FALL OF A PILLAR - DAD'S DEATH

1995 was a very negative year. I worked in Cremona and lived in San Donato (Milan). I had to get up at 5.30 a.m. to drive to the construction site and, while trying the iridology treatment, I got up as early as at 3.00 a.m. My Dad got sick and died after some terrible labor and being left alone by the healthcare system. I tried another CH treatment, as I will describe later on, which contributed to further reducing sleep, while my disorder got worse and worse. My life was characterized by unsustainable stressors.

Talking with Dad, who had already been sick for a while (he suffered from continuous severe back pain, had been diagnosed with hernia and operated, and his general practitioner told him it was age-related pain), we considered using pranotherapy.

Dad used to say: "Since you're here in Milan, and you have the opportunity, why don't you give a try to pranotherapy?"

Translated by Laura Monti – Milan (Italy)

I turned to a pranotherapist who had taken care of my mother. He seemed very capable and had become the president of Italian pranotherapists.

I tried to have him treat me with pranotherapy. It was quite expensive and hardly sustainable for me. Securing his services was quite hard: he didn't make appointments, you just went there and waited for your turn with other people.

Meanwhile one night, as I got home, I heard Dad complaining while taking a bath, unable to move inside the bathtub because of back pain. As I got in, I saw him sitting still. I was not persuaded and thought, "It can't be age-related pain or the hernia he was operated for months ago" (as his GP claimed). I helped him out and took him to the ER unit of the San Donato hospital.

There, I was called in to talk. As I sensed from the looks of the doctors, the situation was serious. They told me, "Your Dad's spine is full of metastases, he must be hospitalized and treated immediately." I did not tell dad, and only mentioned bone decalcification, a disorder related to osteoporosis.

This was the start of an outrageous story of Italian health care for a man who had never needed it, but who had paid contributions for more than forty years!

Translated by Laura Monti – Milan (Italy)

At the hospital, they looked for a suitable place to move him to. There were no free bed places in San Donato, and no hospitals contacted by the ER doctors had vacancies. Just imagine, who would be happy to treat a 68-year-old man full of metastases? He lay on a stretcher in the ER unit of the San Donato hospital for two or three days, while no vacancy could be found in any hospitals in Milan. I took charge, and some friends helped me find a bed place for him in Sondalo, in the upper Valtellina region, where he could have surgery to remove some of those metastases and relieve the spine compressions that caused him so much pain.

After surgery, through friends and acquaintances I managed to find him a place in the oncology unit at the Niguarda hospital in Milan, where he had radiotherapy to slow down the tumor's progression. I won't go into all the details of the troubles we suffered and the arguments I went through. Troubles with the doctors, troubles due to the lack of support from social services, troubles that often characterize Italian health care when dealing with old people with a limited life expectancy. After radiotherapy, one day they told me they had to discharge Dad without notice.

I was astonished. He needed a wheelchair, a reclining bed, someone to take care of him at home, to feed him and help him

Translated by Laura Monti – Milan (Italy)

evacuate, change his diaper, etc. and I worked in Cremona. I left early in the morning and returned in the evening.

I turned to Caritas to have a paid nurse at home on a 24/7 basis and to the geriatric unit of the San Donato hospital, which arranged for a daily visit by a very well-trained male nurse that helped him satisfy his needs.

Things got slowly worse, the metastases spread to the abdomen and stomach, which should be emptied mechanically to prevent from bursting. I took him to the Melegnano hospital, where I received help, they emptied his stomach and hospitalized him again. Dad took eight doses of morphine a day, but was still screaming from pain, he had lost his mind, but held on because he had a strong heart.

Whenever his mind was clear, he asked me to be buried in Morbegno, his hometown, and I reassured him, "Don't worry Dad, I'll take care of that". That was the end, it was only a matter of time, but he continued to suffer terribly because his heart did not give up. I decided to take him home with an automated morphine pump. I decided on my own (without asking my sister), after he told me he wished to die, to speed up the morphine pump as much as possible. His heart collapsed and he stopped suffering as he passed away. He let out his death rattle while I was holding his head in my hands. I was with him to the last second. As I write this, tears run down my face and I feel the

Translated by Laura Monti – Milan (Italy)

same sorrow, but it's nothing compared to the way I felt back then. I had to make this choice for his sake, I know it's illegal, it's murder according to the law, but the love for my Dad reached far beyond any law written by man! This happened from March to September 1995.

Back to pranotherapy, I was treated even while Dad was hospitalized at Niguarda. My typical day was a nightmare: I woke up at 5.30 a.m., drove to the construction site in Montodine to face my working day, finished at 6.00 p.m. and returned to San Donato, took my bike – my Tenerè – and went to see Dad at Niguarda, spent a couple of hours with him and Annalisa, **my girlfriend who has always been there for me at those sad times,** and took him around for a while on a wheelchair. I left Niguarda, had a pizza, and went to the pranotherapist, approximately around 9.00 p.m. I waited for my turn and returned home between 1.00 and 3.00 a.m. Then I woke up at 5.30 a.m. to start a new day.

I can say for sure that stress was my constant companion, I suffered a lot, and turned my anger into the strength I needed to go on. If I think about it now, I don't know how I managed!

While continuing my pranotherapy sessions, I talked with the pranotherapist, asked for explanations and a diagnosis. I hadn't told him I had a right-side CH, I never said on which side, and he claimed I had several problems: I had an energy imbalance, I had

Translated by Laura Monti – Milan (Italy)

problems with my stomach, and this imbalance lead to severe right-side headaches! He claimed I had an extraordinary amount of energy in my body which I couldn't handle or convey, and it was discharged against me causing pain!

He tried to take a Kyrian electro-photograph, which I still have, certifying that I had the characteristics required of a first-level pranotherapist, but still needed to rebalance energy. He offered me a course to become a pranotherapist, which implied a significant cost and an equally significant commitment.

I no longer knew what to believe and what to do. I should have left my work to attend the course, and could hardly pay for it: with the high cost of Imigran® and of caring for Dad, I was almost broke. I also thought it was just a strategy to sell me the course. In short, I didn't know what to think any more, I was almost drained, if not drained altogether, I was worried about Dad and about my labor contract that was about to end, and feared they would move me to some far-away location so that I could no longer be near him. Indeed, the pranotherapy sessions had no effect on the progression of CH (even if the pranotherapist claimed that my lifestyle could not help me improve). In short, I decided to stop, not to take the course, and to devote to my work and to Dad.

Translated by Laura Monti – Milan (Italy)

ODD EXPERIENCES TO CONSIDER

While I was having pranotherapy, I had odd experiences. The pranotherapist was building an appliance, which I then bought, that influenced the brain with electromagnetic fields and served different purposes depending on frequency and intensity. He claimed that our brain generates electromagnetic fields of different frequencies depending on the type of thoughts and emotions, and that these fields were more intense in pranotherapists than in other people. For training purposes, he made me try several times a game he had requested to design: it was a computer horse race, where my horse was connected with me via a helmet and received the electromagnetic fields generated by my brain depending on my mood and thoughts. In short, I could influence my horse's speed according to how I managed to control my mood and thoughts. The more I could relax and no longer think, the faster my horse ran. It worked, I tested it. He was a forerunner, because today's allopathic medicine uses electromagnetic fields to influence the brain. Depression is one of the disorders it addresses by stimulating the muted brain regions.

Translated by Laura Monti – Milan (Italy)

THE INFLUENCE OF EMOTIONAL SHOCKS ON CH

After my father's death, I was relocated to another construction site at Pieve a Nievole, near Pistoia, Tuscany, and never saw the pranotherapist again.

Pranotherapy had not succeeded in removing my attacks, I will never know why, even if that man had "powers" he had shown me in various circumstances. I also abandoned the pranotherapy approach – another failure, I was at a loss, I suffered continuously, CH never subsided, I was tired of only drawing some satisfaction from my stressful work, I hated my life and continued to consider suicide. *"When it comes, I'll jump down a very high building, so that I will enjoy the excitement of flying and promptly die without pain."*

After Dad's death, however, I had no attacks for about a fortnight and immediately noticed this strange phenomenon: I didn't understand, instead of getting worse because of my sorrow, the beast was giving me a break! Odd, after Dad's death I felt the earth shaking under my feet. Dad was a very strong pillar in my life, an example to follow, a very good man, strong, fair, with the sound principles and ideas you hardly see today – **a true life leader**. When I had serious problems he was my reference

Translated by Laura Monti – Milan (Italy)

point, my support, the one who knew how to help me face the worst challenges.

Dad was gone, and I was 26. I FELT SO LONELY, at a loss, abandoned. I suffered a lot, and my CH vanished. At first I didn't know why, but now I know: **I had been through a massive emotional shock!**

NEW TREATMENTS AND EXPERIENCES

In Tuscany, headache was treated at a headache center based on the method of Professor Sicuteri. I think it was at the Careggi hospital in Florence. I got in touch, explained my case, and they immediately granted me an appointment, skipping the waiting lists. They gave priority to cluster headache in the acute phase vs. other cases. Finally something positive, not too common at those times; other cutting-edge headache centers do the same now.

I was allocated to doctor Pietrini, who listened to me for a long time, prescribed an exam – pupillometry – and confirmed the CH diagnosis. I don't remember whether he also prescribed me lithium as a prophylactic treatment, but he also gave me a new medication, Deseril®, alongside a symptomatic drug, Diidergot® injections (a vasoconstrictor) to replace Imigran®.

Translated by Laura Monti – Milan (Italy)

After a while I started to feel better. Deseril® seemed to be effective, the attacks did not vanish, but decreased significantly in number, and I spent more often the day with none.

On the other hand, Diidergot® didn't seem to be very effective. Sometimes it managed to stop the attack, but most of the times it didn't, and I continued to take Imigran® when I sensed an attack was coming.

After a few months of peace compared to my previous conditions, I had chronic CH, and that was bad.

I was highly stimulated at work. My activity was organized differently, it was about building natural gas pipelines on the hills of Pistoia, but most of it didn't take place directly, it was subcontracted. This brought a significant change. I liked this site much better than the previous ones because of the surroundings, because of relationships with the subcontractors, and because I could leverage on my previous experience.

My work at Pieve a Nievole only lasted a few months though, and so did the improvement of my CH, because then I was relocated to the construction site of San Martino Valle Caudina, Campania, and Deseril® was unfortunately removed from the market. I understand that this medication was obtained from an ergot derivative, a hallucinogenic molecule, and was classified as a harmful drug because of certain side effects. The fact is it was

Translated by Laura Monti – Milan (Italy)

removed from the market, whatever the reason, and I went on with lithium alone.

If you want to try Deseril®, I found out it is still on sale in the City of San Marino, as well as in Switzerland. I can tell you I heard that some CH sufferers got benefits from this medication. However, tell your doctor, because it may have side effects.

Around 1997, the then Minister of Health Rosi Bindi moved Imigran® to class A, which means it was 100% reimbursable. God bless her, I don't know what she did for better or for worse in her mandate as minister of health, but this change of class of Imigran® meant a huge saving for me and for others!

In 1997 my life had become utterly unsustainable. I had lost faith in doctors and health care, took lithium without controlling blood levels, continued to inject Imigran® into my arms and legs, yet had attacks every day all year round. Only occasionally I had none for two or three days, and I felt as strong as a lion, I was overjoyed, I deluded myself into thinking that the beast was taking a break. In those two or three days I recharged my batteries at the speed of light, my mood changed to positive, but then the illusion vanished because the beast returned to bite and ravage me.

Translated by Laura Monti – Milan (Italy)

STRANGE BUT TRUE: A CALCIUM CHANNEL BLOCKER FOR PROPHYLAXIS – VERAPAMIL

At that time I was working at the S. Martino Valle Caudina construction site in Campania and had excellent working relations with my foreman. He saw my pitiful conditions and tried to convince me to visit another headache center. I told him my story of failures with doctors and medications. I was depressed, really very sick, and it was all doom and gloom for me. By insisting and making me think that new treatments could have been discovered, he nevertheless convinced me to try.

I decided to wait for the first welding line (the main phase of pipeline construction) to be completed, then started looking for a good headache center. I found the Mondino center in Pavia, headed by Professor Nappi. I wrote him a very assertive letter asking for help, and was proposed hospitalization in response.

At Mondino, the chronic CH diagnosis was confirmed after a number of tests to exclude secondary migraine, i.e. a migraine due to some external causes, such as an arterial occlusion or the like. I was proposed a confirmation test with trinitrin but, given my past experience, I firmly refused!

I had x-rays, carotid doppler, and a pain tolerability test (too high!). All regular, except for a small nodule on the thyroid which was deemed worthy of a check.

Translated by Laura Monti – Milan (Italy)

On that occasion I found out about the existence of **verapamil,** which I was immediately prescribed! I read the medication's leaflet, and got the idea they were crazy to prescribe this drug, but no, they were right: within a few weeks my CH gradually faded away, then vanished.

Great, I couldn't believe it, I felt as strong as a lion. Marco, my foreman, had been right, it had been a good thing to go to Mondino. I remember a lovely creature at Mondino, doctor Martignoni. I remember her for her sweetness when she approached patients. I immediately made arrangements to have needle aspiration from the thyroid nodule they had found in Pavia and, while waiting for histological testing, I returned to work at the San Martino Valle Caudina construction site.

I had returned to work free from the attacks and with an immense gratitude towards my foreman, who had insisted I sought hospitalization. Meanwhile I received the results of my test: undefined, because the test failed and I had to repeat it. I hesitated, because I was very busy with my work and thought, "I'll take the test again when I stop for the Christmas holidays, surely it must be a cyst, like those I had already removed years ago from my face and neck". That was in September 1997.

One day, when I was at the construction site, CH returned despite I was still taking verapamil, and gradually increased, but was not so devastating. I got attacks almost every day, and every

Translated by Laura Monti – Milan (Italy)

now and then even several times a day. I suffered so much that I resumed frequent use of Imigran®. At that point I scheduled a check to find out what was going on. I was examined and, in short, my dose of verapamil was increased. This gave me temporary benefits, but not respite because, as with the previous dose, after a while CH got worse and the dose was no longer effective to prevent the attacks, but just to mitigate them. As a consequence, the dose had to be increased! That was the start of my drug resistance to verapamil.

A CANCER WAS ALL I NEEDED! BUT EVERY CLOUD HAS A SILVER LINING, AND I GET A NEW CONFIRMATION

I was then relocated to the Comiso (Ragusa) construction site in Sicily, a place where I felt very uncomfortable for a number of work-related problems. The Christmas holidays came at last and I returned to Milan. I remembered the failed test and arranged for a new needle aspiration at the Niguarda hospital from the thyroid nodule I had been diagnosed in Pavia. I had the test and left for Sicily to continue my work while waiting for the result.

After a few days I received a phone call from my cousin Clara, who is a doctor at Niguarda. I hadn't heard from and seen her for years, not least because my way of life always kept me away

Translated by Laura Monti – Milan (Italy)

from home, and this call promptly aroused some concern. I had already figured everything out and said to her: "Clara, are you going to tell me I have cancer?".

Unfortunately this was the case: I had a medullar carcinoma in my thyroid and Clara told me I had to return immediately to have my thyroid removed. The carcinoma was not of the most dangerous type, but the development of metastases would have made things much more serious.

I was very determined, I left everything behind in Sicily (rented house, suitcases, clothes, etc.), including my car, and made arrangements to return immediately to Milan, but I told everyone: "Don't worry, I'll kill it and come back," and so I did!!!

I was admitted to the Carati endocrinology unit at Niguarda. There was a medical staff, but the doctor in charge of me was a Ms. Riolo, a lady characterized by great humanity. You could see she had experienced sorrow in her life, because she was great at interacting with patients and was very sweet. I learned to love her very much, too bad she's no longer there, she retired.

Anyway, at the hospital I was very worried about CH and kept pestering the doctors to get Imigran® (which was not available in that unit). I was scared, not so much for surgery or cancer – I was as strong as a lion in that respect – as because I had to withdraw from verapamil to have surgery! It was a nightmare for me,

Translated by Laura Monti – Milan (Italy)

because at the hospital they told me they couldn't give me more than two vials of Imigran® a day, as stated in the leaflet. That was my fear, my worst fear – that my beast would return as bad as ever.

There is something funny, though: despite withdrawing from verapamil, I didn't have any attacks, and this continued for some time, because I stayed in hospital for three to four weeks.

Once again (but I was unaware of this at that time) the shock for my ordeal was keeping my CH at bay!!!

It was a nice adventure, my surgery was repeatedly postponed because transplants had priority and I kept looking for something to do to pass the time. I helped the nurses in charge of elderly patients. I helped Adelmo, an old man I had grown particularly fond of. I drove the nurses crazy because I teased them and made jokes. I would walk around the hospital with a laser pointer (they were not very popular and quite unknown at that time) focusing on the nurses' asses, on the tables in the cafeteria while they were having their meals, and they showered me with questions when they saw that little light! Then, in time, they got to know me and sometimes came to me for help with this and that.

I was quite strong and very upbeat, because CH was leaving me alone until, once I was moved to the surgery unit, after my

Translated by Laura Monti – Milan (Italy)

operation was postponed to give priority to transplants, I saw my five fellow-patients in our six-bed room die!!! I had a harsh argument with the chief of surgery and was finally operated. After a few days in hospital and a few of recovery at home I returned to work. The operation had been more complicated than expected, my parathyroid glands were also removed and one was experimentally re-grafted into the neck; my vocal cords were scraped off and I had laterocervical dissection because of lymph node involvement.

When I returned to the construction site I had no voice and slammed my fists on the table to talk with and be listened to by the foreman, because he had no sympathy for my communication difficulties, but except for that and a number of other challenges at work, I had the usual problem – CH had returned and was causing me troubles.

Time went by, I finished my work at the construction site and meanwhile the company was in hardships. Ground assembly activities in Italy were discontinued and unemployment benefits were applied for. I saw many of my co-workers resort to unemployment benefits and, once back at my office in Milan and far from the dismissed ground assembly sites, I began to worry.

Translated by Laura Monti – Milan (Italy)

ARDUOUS WORK AND CH EXACERBATION - A NEW ADMISSION TO A NEW FACILITY

In the light of what you read at the end of the previous chapter, my foreman told me that, if I wanted to avoid any risk of redundancy, I had to agree to work at sea installations, which is the same as building natural gas / oil pipelines, but laid on the sea bottom, as well as assembling modules to support drilling rigs. These activities are defined as arduous work! Given the situation, I agreed to that, although at that time in my life I was supposed to slow down and seek the advice of a psychologist, being further destabilized by that cancer story. I said to myself, "CH is ok, but what about cancer at 28? What am I doomed for?".

I started working on the D.B. Crawler, a non-powered offshore vehicle operating at that time in the 1999 Adriatic Sea campaign. The situation on board was very poor in terms of safety, and I had to take a firm stance on many aspects that needed to be adjusted and improved. I had to use all my energy and my know how to manage, over about six months, to change the situation on this offshore vehicle, but the positive thing at work was that I achieved my goal. I implemented an on-board safety training program, end-of-month paperwork was duly produced, regular meetings on safety were held before starting any activities, we

Translated by Laura Monti – Milan (Italy)

made abandon-ship drills and practiced people rescuing, etc. In short, things had significantly improved since I first got there.

Life on board was very difficult. I worked 12 hours a day on daily shifts, resting and recreational space was virtually non-existent. I used to stroll on the heliport to relieve tension, where I was forced to inhale dioxin discharges from the rudimentary waste-disposal cauldron located on the bridge, and spent the rest of my free time reading.

The main problem was sleeping. I couldn't sleep, partly because of the noise of the machinery and the pile driver, and partly because one change of the workers' shifts took place during my sleeping hours, and the Filipinos and Malaysians made a hell of a mess that kept me awake.

High levels of stress at work and lack of sleep had affected the number of attacks and I had an average of three to four per day despite the prophylactic treatment. I had to involve the commander to get Imigran® vials through the shipping agency, because the supplies I had taken on board were not enough.

My life was a real torture. I was absolutely unhappy and continued to consider suicide as the only way to freedom. I kept talking to everyone about my illness, as if to prepare them for a possible attack. I was afraid to do anything if I didn't have the Imigran® shots with me. I had become one with Imigran®. Even

Translated by Laura Monti – Milan (Italy)

at home, I never even went out for bread without a shot in my pocket! I was really scared.

After about six months working on the D.B. Crawler I returned to Milan in terrible conditions and asked my medical office where I could turn to try to mitigate CH. I was told to seek help from the San Raffaele neurology unit at Ville Turro. I called, explained my case, and was immediately admitted. That was in 2000.

The first approach provided for cortisone, which removed my attacks for a while, plus oxygen and Imigran® for any residual crises. Finally, prophylactic verapamil again. During my stay in hospital I enjoyed some peace, I could finally take care of myself, and cortisone gave me some respite from the attacks. At last, I needed that!

At that time, an antiepileptic had also been included in the prophylactic treatment and had proved effective in some CH sufferers. I had to reach the effective dose gradually in order to take it, but suffered several circulation disorders in the process, particularly in the legs, and had to discontinue it. However I believe that the fact an antiepileptic can be effective on CH shows that there is indeed electric brain hyperactivity in CH sufferers.

After being discharged, I spent about three years working at my company's headquarters in San Donato Milanese.

Translated by Laura Monti – Milan (Italy)

A DREAM COMES TRUE AND THE INTERFERENCE OF EMOTIONAL SHOCKS ON CH IS CONFIRMED – O.U.C.H. Italy Onlus

In those three years I could finally get in touch through the internet with another CH sufferer – Riccardo Pentenero. We talked to each other, spent hours on the phone, and he told me he had already met other sufferers via the internet. That's when contacts with other fellow-sufferers! We resolved to meet and we first did at the premises of a lovely creature called Piera Ravazzoli.

It was a dazzling meeting, to say the least, a unique emotion mixed with overwhelming joy. After the first meeting we decided to found OUCH Italy Onlus as a branch of OUCH USA, but significantly that strong emotion that pervaded my body like a shock, albeit positive, granted me a few days of respite at a time when I used to have multiple daily attacks. **Shocks are effective – whether positive or negative.** That was in 2001.

Five of us founded the association, but one vanished right away and we virtually never heard from him again. OUCH began its activity with the launch of the forum for CH sufferers, which soon became a reference point for many, including non-members.

Translated by Laura Monti – Milan (Italy)

The first OUCH meeting was then organized. People met at different locations and discussed together, while also pursuing some of the objectives set by the association.

Once again the first meeting aroused a very strong emotion and I enjoyed a few more days of respite. Even more significant about the fact that respite occurs downstream to positive or negative shocks is that this also happened to other CH sufferers: some of them joined the forum and, by discussing with us, finding a reference point, being able to feel welcomed and understood by other people that suffered from the same illness and to pour out their tragedy, experienced either an improvement or partial remission. **This further confirmed the influence of emotional shocks on our illness.** We at OUCH became aware of this phenomenon, which we started monitoring through all the new entries into the forum and subsequent meetings with the new CH sufferers we met. *Shocks turned out to have a positive impact in most cases.*

Of course I didn't enjoy the same effect after the second meeting, because the emotion was no longer as strong as it used to be at first, but I observed that the same happened to newcomers!

Translated by Laura Monti – Milan (Italy)

PERSONAL RESEARCH INTO THE COMMON TRAITS OF CH SUFFERERS

Since the founding of the association, I embarked on an individual and personal activity, as I mentioned in the introduction, implemented through an analysis of people in one-to-one meetings. In fact I had realized that people in the forum sort of wore a "mask," were not utterly honest, did not open up completely, and did not display their most sensitive traits. The reason was clear – the forum was public and discouraged full disclosure.

At those meetings I looked for potential common traits and found some that reassured me and helped me understand that most of the things that happened to me were consequences of CH. Almost all sufferers had sudden temperature changes during and after the attacks; many reported neurovegetative imbalances during the clusters; many had a rather strong sexual attitude and libido; many said that they first suffered from CH **following events that can be classified as post-traumatic stress:** raped girls, people that grew up with an alcohol-addicted father that beat their mother, that never went past the death of a family member or breaking up with their partner, that went through psychedelic drug use/abuse. In short, a broad range of events that caused a shock to the concerned people (of course,

Translated by Laura Monti – Milan (Italy)

no one spoke about these facts in the forum, too personal to be dealt with in public).

The approach to this kind of events was obviously extremely subjective. In fact some people do not make a fuss if left by their partner and go on almost as if nothing had happened, while others experience the event with great sorrow, as an insurmountable trauma that has scarred their life. The same is true for bereavement or other types of shocks. This is also extremely subjective. You can try to perform an introspective investigation into yourself to see if your CH started after an event that was <u>PARTICULARLY EMOTIONAL FOR YOU</u>, one you never managed to get past. This aspect did not emerge in some people, either because it didn't happen or because the concerned individual was still unaware.

However, I carried out this investigation for about ten years and it helped me move forward in my studies – not scientific but based on real life – on the illness.

Another characteristic I found I share with many other CH sufferers is meteoropathy, i.e. sensitivity to sudden weather changes. That's quite telling. In practice it happens that, facing sudden drops in temperature or sudden peaks of humidity during a cluster, we sufferers experience an exacerbation of our attacks, and if no cluster is under way, it may be triggered. When I used to drive home from southern Italy or back and a storm was

Translated by Laura Monti – Milan (Italy)

approaching, I even happened to gradually feel the attack coming, as if I could sense the storm's electricity in the air, and then fading when the storm was over.

This clearly shows that, when the weather changes, our neuroendocrine system is set in motion to react to the resulting stress, and probably fails to promote the necessary adjustment. In other words, a drop in temperature acts as an environmental stressor for our body because it requires an adjustment of our body temperature control system that happens to originate in the hypothalamus!!! We may have greater difficulty at dealing with the stressors – of any nature – acting on us. They are environmental in this example, but they can also be related to our work, emotional, or of any other origin. *I understand that the reaction to stressors is always a basic hypothalamic response.*

On average, I also identified some shared characteristics of our personality. Almost all the CH sufferers I met were hyperactive and hyper-busy people, who usually had great responsibility at work and, if they didn't, generated such responsibility through their approach and attitude. These people were very intense, serious, and emotional about their life; some tended to be perfectionists, certainly not superficial; they brooded a lot, perhaps too much, on everything. I never met a calm, peaceful, and quiet CH sufferer and, if there is one, he or she is the exception that proves the rule. It is not clear whether this is a consequence or a contributing cause, an intrinsic characteristic of CH.

Another identified characteristic of CH was that it seems to strike when relaxing. In other words, night attacks occur during sleep, but daytime ones seem to occur at times of lower tension. An attack hardly ever occurs when you have to carry out a stressful activity, but once the activity is completed and the time comes to relax, you most likely get the attack. Likewise, if you are working hard and then go on vacation and suddenly relax, CH explodes and gets worse. As I went on vacation, I often happened to change from my pre-vacation lifestyle: I slept longer and I suddenly relaxed. By doing so, my head exploded, the number and frequency of the attacks soared. Later, as I realized this, I learned to avoid sudden relax and to enjoy it gradually. For example, if I usually got up at 6.30 a.m. to go to work, on vacation I had to get up not later than at 7.00 a.m., because if I overslept I would get an attack. I woke up for a few days at 7.00 a.m., for a few days at 7.30 a.m. and so on. Over time I would gradually wake up later and later.

This obviously did not concern sleep only, but also day life. Therefore I had to carry out activities that would keep me up and going, and not too much relaxed.

Translated by Laura Monti – Milan (Italy)

To sum it up, the transition between tension and relaxation should be gradual to avoid feeding the beast, because any sudden change, even if for the better, is by definition a stressor!

TIME GOES BY AND DESPAIR MAKES ME DO ODD THINGS

Meanwhile, my CH was always there and by then chronic and drug resistant for a long time. I was definitely disabled. I fancied starting my own business by establishing a company that dealt with safety at work, but was afraid ... considering the situation, I lacked the courage!

I approached a homeopath who gave me strange medicines, granules to be dissolved under the tongue. I complied with treatment, but got no benefit – another frustrated hope.

Desperation was part of me. I heard about a sort of witchdoctor based in Milan, an old man that could provide diagnoses and prognoses solely based on used underwear. I was really in despair and ... well ... I tried this option. I took him my undershirt, queued up patiently waiting for my turn, and was then told I was stressed and had to treat my disorder with a cream I had to prepare myself with castor oil. I did so because I no longer knew

Translated by Laura Monti – Milan (Italy)

what else I could try. You may think I was crazy, but despair plays tricks and makes you cling to any hope you may have. However, the treatment did not give me any benefit and, of course, my emotional sphere was increasingly frustrated. I was angry with the whole world and all the things around me – I was definitely in a frenzy.

SOMETIMES PERSISTENCE AND COMMITMENT ARE REWARDED

There was something positive though: OUCH Italy had been established and had radically changed my perception of CH, because then I no longer felt lonely. In psychological terms, this was a major step forward, also shared by dozens of CH sufferers that later interacted with us. **At that time my greatest aspiration was to understand CH, to gain a deep insight of it, and to find the best solutions for myself and for others!**

Managing the association was no easy task, though. On one hand only two or three people were usually active, and there is not much few people can do. On the other, while we continued to try to also involve those that were not on the board of directors, hardly anyone came forward to help.

Translated by Laura Monti – Milan (Italy)

Reconciling work engagements, family, and health – by then in poor conditions – with the association's commitments and the daily running of the forum was not easy. The mutual interface among CH sufferers with different subjective traits was another obstacle to pursuing the objectives of the association, although the spirit that united us at the outset, in the early years, was so strong it could meet all these challenges. Then we managed to do something good also from the institutional point of view. We attended an event at Palazzo Marino in Rome, organized by the Dossetti Association on rare diseases, where I had the opportunity to describe the characteristics of CH, its severity and its rarity, to senators and deputies. The aim was to arouse awareness of the existence of this illness, which even general practitioners and neurologists often ignored. We got in touch with AIC (Associazione Italiana Cefalalgici, the Italian association of headache sufferers) and the scientific community, in the historical premises of the Besta Institute in Milan, with whom we collaborated to explain the seriousness of this disease to the regional authorities of Lombardy. This excellent work was aimed at obtaining the acknowledgement of disability for severe CH sufferers. The goal was then achieved and today CH is recognized as a disabling illness in Lombardy. However for this work we must sincerely thank a legendary member of AIC (whose name I will not mention for privacy reasons), head of the Lombardy

Translated by Laura Monti – Milan (Italy)

region, for his commitment and his great work. He was a tough man that never gave up!

As part of our activities, we attended an OUCH USA meeting in Vancouver, Canada. This too was an extraordinary experience: even with the Americans, we seemed to have known each other for a long time, the illness we shared was a strong glue that immediately resulted into a close friendship and great mutual sympathy. The meeting also discussed the use of hallucinogenic molecules such as LSD and psilocybe, and former users were nice-looking people, regular family fathers, who certainly did not use those drug for recreational purposes, but to leverage on their true efficacy. Indeed, I remember they stressed that the effective dose was much lower than the recreational one. In fact I was keen on knowing whether they were drug addicted, I wanted to look into their eyes to understand. At those meetings, oxygen was massively used to counter the attacks, something that in Italy had not yet caught on.

We attended several conventions on headaches in view of spreading the news of our association, but in fact it was a small association, with few members, and completely penniless, so that we could not even consider investments of any kind. Just think that, whenever we attended an event, we all paid travel and accommodation expenses out of our own pockets!

Translated by Laura Monti – Milan (Italy)

On those occasions we also got in touch with the scientific community and met outstanding people and CH experts, such as Professor Bussone, Doctor Leone, Doctor Frediani, Doctor Cerbo, Doctor Tanzini, etc. Over time, these figures were invited to the OUCH meetings, which then took on a more professional character. I remained involved in the association with an active role for more than ten years, then I left for force majeure.

DO YOU THINK I TRIED AGAIN OR GAVE UP?

On a beautiful day I heard about plantar digital pressure performed in Milan, which was said to be effective even against CH. So I decided to go for this umpteenth attempt.

I went once a week to a clinic near the main Railway Station to submit to this type of pressure, then combined with hypnosis. All of this, of course, for a fee! It was quite painful: the operator used a tool to press a point on my big toe and caused excruciating pain throughout the session. I was given odd explanations about what he was doing, allegedly breaking crystals that were generated in that "trigger" area, but honestly I never quite understood. I insisted a lot with this approach combined with hypnosis and, whether it was by chance or thanks to this treatment, things improved for a while, but then reverted

Translated by Laura Monti – Milan (Italy)

to the original situation: medications – Isoptin® 720 mg/day and Imigran® as needed, and an average of two to three attacks per day notwithstanding. I occasionally took cortisone to enjoy some time off from this persistent suffering.

But I made more attempts, I didn't give up, and heard about a naturopath in Milan, with a clinic near via Melchiorre Gioia. He used naturopathy, which I heard was quite effective. He treated patients with oxygen/ozone therapy, homeopathy, herbal medicine, Ayurvedic medicine, hydrocolon therapy, and chromotherapy. Who knows, maybe they could be effective! I made an appointment, went there and got a strange diagnosis through bioelectronic medicine, a branch of natural medicine that makes use of electronic diagnostic tools, capable to translate changes in the electrical resistance of the skin into measurable electrical signals. I submitted to this diagnostic approach and, in response, I got a prescription to read verses of the Bible several times a day! I didn't understand, I thought he would apply some of the above natural therapies to me, but instead I found myself reading verses of the Bible several times a day. I went back home in amazement and started to do so for a few days, then I felt so stupid that I stopped this so-called treatment and didn't return, also considering that such sessions were quite expensive!

Translated by Laura Monti – Milan (Italy)

OF COURSE I STILL NEED TO WORK TO EARN A LIVING

From 2003 to 2005 I returned to work in construction sites and to travel around Italy, first to the military facility of Perdasdefogus in the province of Nuoro, Sardinia (like, "let's get some military radiations"), where I was in charge of a special project called TAP (Trasporto Alta Pressione, or High Pressure Transport), then several times in Gela, Sicily, where I had been in charge of the P2bis line (a project banned by the judiciary), the reconstruction of the Foranea Dam – both inside the Gela Petrochemical plant (some pollution is just good for your health ☺) – and the LGTS (Libya Gas Transmission System) project.

With this last job, required to import natural gas from Libya, I reverted to very high levels of stress and fear. The organization was very poor, most of the time activities took place on a 24-hour basis, and I was the only resource in charge of security, so that I had to cover both work shifts, day and night. To cut it short, I was suffering a work overload.

Then there was an accident with a mafia family from Gela, which I am not going to describe for cautionary reasons. The clash we had was such that they threatened to take my girls away from me!

Translated by Laura Monti – Milan (Italy)

This aroused a huge amount of anxiety, I couldn't sleep and was always on the lookout lest something would happen to me. At that hell of a time, I suffered as many as 8 attacks a day.

Following a series of fortuitous events, I approached meditation and discovered Osho Rainesch, an oriental life coach whose many books I later read.

I found the meditation practice more effective than medications. Benzodiazepines didn't work for sleeping, but after an hour of meditation I fell asleep like a baby. Osho's meditation and teachings made me aware of how wrong my way of living was, my way of struggling against the wrong things, of countering CH, of constantly living at high speed without ever enjoying some me-time. It made me understand how necessary it was to start slowing down.

PRACTICE MAKES PERFECT

That is how I slowly began to try to change my lifestyle.

The first step – which you too need to take, if you haven't yet – is to **accept your illness.** You must accept to be sick with CH, simply accept it deep down in your heart, and then live accordingly.

The second step I learned to take was to stop thinking all the time about CH as if it were something that was part of me

Translated by Laura Monti – Milan (Italy)

twenty-four hours a day, and rather only face and address it at the time of the attacks. In other words, chronic CH sufferers tend to keep talking about their illness and saying they always have a headache. But this cannot be true: even if the attacks occur every day, they are limited in time and, though ravaging, thank God they only last sixty to forty minutes on average. This is to say that our psychological relation with our illness does not continue throughout the day, but is only limited to the duration of the attacks. We should try to see the attack as a parenthesis in our life that contains all our pain and anger, but when the parenthesis is closed our life, which is not just made of suffering, continues its course. We must learn to live in the present! Easier said than done, but continuous training helps!

I found meditation very helpful to change my approach to CH. My anger subsided, my suffering decreased, and my quality of life improved. By that time I had also learned to brood less by using less of my brain and to slow down with my body by moving and walking just as slowly, striving to do so consciously and deliberately.

This **hard work** through meditation had a truly unexpected outcome. Chronic CH was still there, maybe with fewer attacks, but in fact I suffered less, and when I did I managed to deal with the suffering. I was changing my attitude towards the illness. THE

Translated by Laura Monti – Milan (Italy)

ILLNESS WAS STILL THE SAME, BUT I WAS CHANGING through hard work, failures, yet great determination.

A NEUROLOGIST I CALL SPECIAL

That was in 2006 and I was still a chronic drug-resistant cluster headache sufferer. Perhaps I had a few more weapons, but still suffered an outrageous number of attacks. By then I had been treated for a few years by Doctor Fabio Frediani, whom I had known for some time. He was the president of AIC and we had worked together towards some goals, such as the acknowledgement of CH as a disability by the Lombardy region. I liked this man very much because he is a wonderful human being, as much as a great neurologist, capable to listen to his patients and – equally important to me – to devote all the necessary time to checks (other than I noticed in many other cases).

I also confronted with him on the **study of the possible causes of cluster headache,** and shared with him some common traits I had observed in the one-to-one work with other CH sufferers I had been engaging in for several years. We were in perfect agreement on one point: **shocks have a direct influence on CH**, whatever their kind.

Translated by Laura Monti – Milan (Italy)

My case was a difficult one that did not respond properly to medications. The variety of options under consideration included DBS (deep brain stimulation), which I had discarded at the outset for the above-mentioned reasons. Having said that, Doctor Frediani asked me whether I had ever experienced a direct drug shock produced with a cortisone bolus. A cortisone bolus is a five-day intravenous infusion of one gram of cortisone per day – a definitely high dose that causes a **drug shock** to the neuroendocrine system. Just to give you a clearer idea, consider that the oral dose of Deltacortene® is a 25mg tablet, then reduced to a 5mg tablet (the drug dose that reaches blood circulation is much lower after oral intake). The intramuscular route produces more limited drug dispersion, compared to the oral route, but not all of the dose reaches the bloodstream because only a share of it is absorbed. Decadron® 4 or 8mg intramuscular injections are generally used. I had never tried the cortisone bolus, and together we decided to go for it in view of possible remission.

I was admitted to the Ponte San Pietro hospital, in the neighborhood of Bergamo, where he worked, and was administered the bolus along with stomach protectors.

CH vanished on day one, but I suffered a number of severe side effects: I was famished, had insomnia, and became very aggressive. My anger tended to come out ever too easily. Thank

Translated by Laura Monti – Milan (Italy)

God I had a clear mind and realized I needed to control my outbursts. One day, early in the morning, a nurse entered my room and woke us up turning on the light and shouting out loud the name of my roommate, who was half deaf. I am one that finds it extremely difficult to wake up, wake-up time is the hardest time of the day for me, when I very often suffer CH attacks and am sensitive to light. I went crazy! I suddenly got up and was about to jump on her and beat her. I even considered throwing her out of the window, but then I realized what was going on with me and left the room to cool down. If I had surrendered to my instinct, I would have killed her!

After some time, I returned to my room and, upon my daily check, told Doctor Frediani to make sure that such methods, such awakenings, be avoided because if on one hand it was wrong to wake up people like that, on the other I was in a special condition and, if I hadn't been able to control myself, I could have had a dangerous and uncontrolled overreaction.

Back to the main issue, the attacks vanished when I had the bolus. I was discharged with a prescription to gradually scale down cortisone and, while I did, I had no attacks. When I stopped taking cortisone I had no more attacks for five days. It seemed it had worked and brought about remission, but no, CH came back... the bolus had only had a temporary effect. Damn, we didn't get the expected results!

Translated by Laura Monti – Milan (Italy)

I naturally reverted to my huge dose of verapamil 720 mg/day, (consider that I weighed about 56Kg), to oral cortisone and Imigran® for the attacks, which continued to appear two or three times a day, with a few occasional days of respite in-between.

Not being satisfied, we thought about another potential shock-generating strategy and Doctor Frediani suggested – if I felt comfortable with it – to try a reverse drug shock, i.e. suddenly stop all medications and take nothing!

Help... I decided to make this one more attempt!

I lived through a nightmare, with continuous attacks. I had an average of two overnight lasting sixty to ninety minutes, which left me devastated... and I went for meditation in pain waiting for them to subside. I applied the techniques I had used before taking up Imigran®, because I didn't even take it, I pressed the trigger points on my head and tried to associate with the pain, to become THE PAIN, in order to try to reduce the perceived suffering. Sometimes I succeeded, but sometimes I didn't. I meditated both in the morning and in the evening to develop stronger motivation, because it was really hard to resist.

After about fifty days of this damned suffering CH vanished as if by magic! I couldn't believe it, one day, two days went by, then three, seven, ten, and still no attacks. I was stunned, but that was it!

Translated by Laura Monti – Milan (Italy)

A CHANGE OF DIRECTION

That was the start of the real transformation of my CH, which would then become a secondary problem for me and allow me to live and enjoy my life, something I couldn't do before.

Unfortunately on June 26, 2006, after twenty-one attack-free days, I had a terrible accident with my motorcycle. It was another shock for me, and a very severe one.

I broke several vertebrae, split my nose, cheekbones and forehead, had three left brain hemorrhages, and crumbled the head of the right humerus to such an extent that I had to have surgery twice, the first to rebuild it and then to remove plates and screws.

In the accident, I lost consciousness and woke up at the hospital. I was forced to lie down for about a month without being able to stand up because of the broken vertebrae, then I started to move wearing a stiff corset. Meanwhile, I had multiple CT scans to monitor the hemorrhages, and on day three they stopped.

I experienced unprecedented events. With a clear mind, I realized I couldn't recognize the people that called me: they said their name and it meant nothing to me – I had lost my memory. I

Translated by Laura Monti – Milan (Italy)

fell into strong reactive depression to the extent that I was moved to a psychiatric unit for treatment.

I still had no CH attacks and this was a great success, a unique success in my CH history, therefore I decided to refuse to take the antidepressants they wanted to prescribe in the psychiatry unit for fear they would interfere at serotonergic level.

The doctor in charge told me that she wouldn't let me go unless I took the medications, but I referred directly to the head physician who, after hearing my story and speaking with Doctor Frediani, understood! However he explained he could not discharge me with persisting severe depression, and I had to do my best to recover and react.

There was a difficult situation in the unit, with serious cases of psychiatric disorders, aggressive people tied to their beds that kept screaming threats, window bars, and one hour outdoor breaks under the nurse's control. I often felt like crying, and then I would hide in the bathroom to calm down and not let the doctors see me, lest they had second thoughts. I was locked up in that unit for a couple of weeks, then I was discharged.

Weeks went by and I still had no attacks. The reverse drug shock had finally been effective, except that its effectiveness had been ascertained for 21 days, because then another shock – caused by the accident – had surely had an impact or had anyway provided an additional input (including the general anesthesia I had for humerus surgery).

I left the hospital and started physical and mental rehab to recovery my memory. I had physical rehab three times a week and daily PC drills, Sony Ericsson memory recovery drills, while at the same time I sought help from a psychologist with an experience in emotional traumas.

In September 2006 I started to suffer annoying day-long left-side migraines that, however, responded to ordinary painkillers. By January, those migraines had changed to the typical characteristics of CH, but their intensity was initially mild and I easily managed them. The problem is that those left-side attacks occurred several times a day, up to three, then slowly became more intense to the extent that they started to affect my life. *Dear me, not again!* When I first had right-side CH, the attacks were also mild and, with that in mind, I started to worry. The good news was that these attacks subsided with high doses of oxygen, which was not the case with the right-side attacks.

After about two months, in March, **I decided to go for a new shock-based approach** and tried psilocybe, a hallucinogenic molecule contained in mushrooms that also grow in Italy.

I got information from the Clusterbuster website, dedicated to this treatment for CH, and embarked on this new experience.

Translated by Laura Monti – Milan (Italy)

On March 3, 2007, and then again on March 09, 2007, I had tea made with about half a gram (a very low dose) of dried mushrooms, and experienced no hallucinogenic or other effects. CH did not vanish, but I only had one daily attack instead of three, and slightly farther apart.

Time went by and the left-side attacks continued, but their intensity had nothing to do with the right-side attacks I had suffered before, which had never reappeared after the reverse drug shock in late May 2006.

These left-side attacks started after the three brain hemorrhages caused by that motorcycle accident on June 26, 2006. Their intensity increased over time, and I occasionally had to go for Imigran®.

By August 2007 the damned right-side attacks were back as bad and strong as ever. I immediately called Doctor Frediani for help and together we decided on an unusual verapamil-based approach that produced some kind of shock to my system, i.e. a daily intake of my effective dose. Verapamil is a drug that is usually administered by gradually increasing the dose over time until it reaches the effective dose, but this time I took my effective dose right away following an ECG check.

CH vanished after two days, but in September 2007, while I was trying to scale down verapamil, it returned on the right side as bad as ever.

At that point I discontinued verapamil, waited a few days for drug clearance, and had a tea made with a high dose – three grams – of dried psilocybe. Please note that I only drank the tea but did not eat the mushrooms, because I was scared by this approach. Thus the absorbed dose was lower than the one I would have taken if I had also consumed the mushrooms.

I still had no hallucinations, but only an altered vision of colors, which looked brighter, a clearer vision of my thoughts, and severe bowel discomfort, including colics and "farts".

Since then the attacks have disappeared, both on the right and on the left. Psilocybe has worked. At first it had turned out ineffective because I had probably used too low a dose.

It was the beginning of a very happy time for me, because after three months I was still CH free! I couldn't believe it, I felt I was living a different life. I slowly regained hope and the fear of the next attack vanished, an anguish that used to oppress my life. I went to work, shopping, eating out, and whatever else, and even though I kept a vial in my car, for cautionary reasons, I did not live in fear anymore and did things without always keeping Imigran® in my pocket. It was another life, another way of living!

Translated by Laura Monti – Milan (Italy)

AFTER PEACE A NEW WAR

Sadly, for some time I had been feeling pain when swallowing coffee, wine, or spicy food and I was being monitored to find out the reason. After more than one year into the investigation phase, I finally had gastroscopy with biopsy.

After the examination, and before the report was ready for pick-up, the hospital called me, which is very unusual, and I understood there was something wrong, so I made an appointment.

At the meeting, when I was told I had a spinocellular carcinoma, I couldn't hold back my tears. In short, I would never be comfortable with my health. I was told how aggressive this cancer is and was explained the need to perform immediate and complex surgery.

In a nutshell, the operation consisted in removing the esophagus, except a section about three centimeters long, together with the branches of the vagus nerve connected thereto. Then the stomach would be extracted, cut, and rebuilt it in the shape of a tube, also removing two arteries out of three, and then connected in the throat in the place of the esophagus!

Translated by Laura Monti – Milan (Italy)

In February 2009 I was admitted to the hospital and had surgery. I spend a few days in the ICU, and can hardly describe the effort I made to hold on and the suffering I was going through. Then, once beyond the most critical moment, I was moved to the in-patient unit.

The post-surgery course was not too good. The connection of the stomach with the remaining esophagus tract in the throat had failed, which meant I was still unable to eat and was fed with a tube from the nose to the stomach for three weeks. It may sound trivial, but that tube hurt like hell. When I spoke it moved and tapped my throat, always in the same place. Over time that part swelled and hurt even with the slightest breathing movement and I got to the point that I could hardly speak.

While in hospital in the post-surgery period my right lung, which had been caused artificial collapse to gain more operating space, did not recover and air had to be drained by inserting a cannula into the clavicle region. This caused an infection with on-going mild fever, and I was prescribed antibiotics.

After a while, when the fever seemed to be fading, I was discharged. On the first day at home I had respiratory distress and after three days I needed oxygen, which I fortunately still had for my CH.

Translated by Laura Monti – Milan (Italy)

I returned to the hospital and was admitted to the lung unit in emergency for severe lung infection from methicillin-resistant bacteria. I had to spend a few more weeks in hospital for i.v. antibiotic therapy and had micro-surgery for subclavicular artery access in order to preserve the veins in the arms. It seemed that lung bursitis housing the bacteria was reluctant to surrender to the antibiotics and the risk was another surgery, this time in the lung. I was very much disturbed by the idea, I was exhausted from all the troubles I had gone through and just didn't want another surgery (not least because the right lung was affected and, although I didn't mention it, I had already suffered a spontaneous pneumothorax on the left I had never recovered from. This had called for removal of the top of the left lung and pleura cautery, and it took about 10 years to regain skin sensitivity at thoracic level and feel no pain when touching). Luckily, the problem was solved and I was discharged.

All the while, CH never occurred either on the right or on the left and this was incredible for me and for my history as a CH sufferer. Repeated shocks continued to influence my CH for the better or for the worse. That was in March 2009.

Months and years went by and CH did not reappear until January 2012, when a very stressful event at work (a work overload and serious criminal liabilities to be managed, without being granted adequate human resources by number and quality, caused me a

Translated by Laura Monti – Milan (Italy)

nervous breakdown, which required in-patient treatment) triggered it again. At first I had left-side attacks that were not as strong as those on the right side and reacted to the use of oxygen, but they were not as mild as they used to be.

I decided to try not to take anything and monitor the course of this left-side CH, and continued using oxygen when at home and Imigran® when away from home, except that in some other cases I just endured the attack.

I went on like this until March, when I called Doctor Frediani to re-consider drug-based prophylaxis. I was instructed to return to verapamil at my effective dose of 720 mg/day, and since it had been a long time since my last ECG check, I also had one.

I took Verapamil as Dr. Frediani had instructed me and within three days the attacks subsided. In the absence of attacks I scaled down verapamil by 120 mg/day every three weeks or so.

In April, while I was in the process of scaling down Isoptin®, CH reappeared, this time on the right, and I was in trouble because oxygen was not effective and the attacks were much more severe. So I decided to revert to Isoptin® 480 mg/day and scale it down more slowly, i.e. 120 mg/day every four attack-free weeks.

Once I stopped Isoptin®, CH left me alone for another two months, then returned and I approached it as follows: when on the left, I tried to control it with Imigran® at the least and only used Isoptin® if it became particularly strong; when on the right, I immediately resorted to Isoptin® because oxygen was not effective to stop it immediately.

The Isoptin®-based approach was very effective because direct intake at the effective dose removed the attacks within about two/three days, then I took off 120mg/day every three or four weeks.

My CH seemed to have a life of its own and to grow undisturbed. However, once we managed to achieve "actual remission" with a succession of shocks, some wanted/sought, others random/accidental, there came another shock (in this case traumatic) on the left (although my CH had started on the right and only occurred on the right). When the attack started on the left it was like one on the right – not too bad, sometimes bearable. If I had known about the use of oxygen – something I didn't at the time – I could have dealt with it without Imigran®, thus avoiding the side effects, etc. CH had also started in the episodic form, and was gradually characterized over time by heavier and heavier clusters (of such a pain intensity and frequency that they gradually called for an increased use of Imigran®).

On the positive side, I now know what it is all about, I am much more informed, and have many more ways to **"wear it down."** However, it is alive, it goes through a phase of gradual worsening and tends to become chronic. In fact I can hardly give up

Translated by Laura Monti – Milan (Italy)

verapamil. It is not yet drug-resistant, I hope it will never be, but verapamil should be scaled down more slowly and the periods of drug-free remission are shrinking.

Time will reveal new things I still don't know, because now I observe and experience my CH with a different mind.

However I must admit that I have still not addressed my left-side CH with all the tools and knowledge I have.

CONCLUSIONS AND PEARLS OF WISDOM

My CH started to change in June 2006 and developed from a chronic, drug-resistant CH, still with two or three attacks a day despite high doses of Isoptin®, to a CH I could keep under control with the right dose of Isoptin®, which didn't cause any more suffering. This also allowed me to stop the vicious cycle established with the ongoing use of Imigran®, which feeds CH and calls for more doses (I repeat, this is my opinion, which I share with many other CH sufferers, but it has no scientific confirmation).

It was a huge success for me that radically changed my life and my lifelong suffering. Today I can go out carefree, without any fear of my beast, confident that it will not make me suffer and that the right dose of Isoptin®, in case of attacks, will control it.

Translated by Laura Monti – Milan (Italy)

This change from my previous condition to the present one, where CH is no longer the number one problem in my life, allowed me to return to live and enjoy life.

The shock-based approach used, sometimes deliberately and sometimes at random, is clearly effective. Other wear-down approaches were obviously attempted over time and influenced the progression of CH. I **first began to accept the illness** and to consider myself a cluster headache sufferer. I accepted this misfortune and reacted accordingly. React accordingly means respect it, do all the things that make it better, and avoid those that make it worse.

I had stopped oversleeping on Saturdays and Sundays, no afternoon naps, no alcohol, I was no longer as stressed as I was when I worked in construction sites, I did meditation and tried to slow down the flow of thoughts, or at least to avoid to cling to it, to keep my emotions a little more under control and not to be "slave to my mind and feelings," but rather be their creator and proactive controller. All this had already turned out beneficial in a CH that was still severe, but somewhat less compared to when I was not that cautious.

To sum it up, shocks had the following effects on my chronic drug-resistant CH: direct drug shocks (cortisone bolus) in 2006 had a true effect, but limited in time. The reverse drug shock of June 2006 produced a 21-day remission, and we don't know how long it would have lasted but for another severe shock I suffered 21 days later due to a bad motorcycle accident. On September 2006 left-side headaches started and developed into CH in less than six months, in January 2007. In March I took two doses of psilocybe that were almost completely ineffective – they only reduced the frequency of the left-side attacks.

In August 2007 CH reappeared on the right and vanished with the verapamil shock, but then, as I scaled down the dose, it returned and I took a 3gr dose of dry psilocybe (I had another severe shock in February 2009), which stopped it until January 2012 when it returned after a traumatic event (another shock).

As mentioned above, I noticed that in most cases CH was triggered by a post-traumatic shock, and more shocks can result into remission.

As you read my story, you can easily see that I enjoyed my first greatest successes in June 2006. **In fact, I went through long periods of remission that I had never experienced before, and at times my CH was absolutely controllable** (an extraordinary change), caused no more fear, and **was no longer strong enough to control, spoil, and destroy my life.** Now I am the one in control, now I can leave home with no vials of Imigran® in my pocket and go to places with loud music, which no longer disturbs me. I can see the light as soon as I wake up without the risk of an attack. I don't get an attack if the temperature

Translated by Laura Monti – Milan (Italy)

suddenly drops. I can drink wine at meals. I can do all these things, and I can hardly believe I can tell you this, **because I am so strongly influenced by my past that I need to give me a pinch to make sure I'm awake as I tell you about my achievements.**

Briefly, my true achievement is my quality of life, which has radically changed with respect to CH. Unfortunately, other health problems have settled in my life: I have troubles eating, sometimes I suffer from a dumping syndrome that triggers post-meal hypoglycemic crises and at times I have severe asthenia, I can hardly lie down and sleep, I endure some small tortures due to the esophageal cancer surgery, but they are nothing compared to the torture of having three attacks of drug-resistant CH per day throughout the year.

I have not been a good patient and I have not been able to deal properly with the CH treatment with the neurologist's support. I say so because I don't want you to make the same mistake. Whenever I noticed a treatment was ineffective or only partially effective, I sought help elsewhere, saw a different neurologist. This is not the right way to go! Ideally, you should find a well-trained neurologist at a reliable headache center acknowledged by the scientific community, and establish a one-to-one mutual relationship to deal with the illness with medications. This allows your neurologist to get to know you, to understand the interaction that medications have with you, the side effects and

Translated by Laura Monti – Milan (Italy)

the beneficial effects. It allows to make the necessary adjustments, to improve the treatments, the drug dosage, the drug combination, the reuse of drugs that did not produce the expected result beforehand – in short, it allows the neurologist to know you over time and to improve your treatments.

If you keep changing, it's like starting over again each time. Feel free to visit several accredited headache centers to find the neurologist you feel you can trust and rely upon, but then try to stay with him or her and be properly monitored. Take note (lest you forget) of the effects of medications, keep a simple headache diary to help the neurologist help you. If your neurologist is a good practitioner, he or she is aware of his/her "mission" in life, which is to help you. If a treatment doesn't work, don't get angry with him/her – I understand you would, but rationally, you cannot put the blame on him/her. A well-trained neurologist is not only capable to administer drugs, but also to put you off them, to make you clear your body from potential drug intoxication. He/she can decide when it's time to stop for hospitalization or a follow-up, but remember he/she is primarily trained on medication use. He/she will hardly tell you to drink a lot of water or do meditation, and so it is always you that have to hold your beast at bay and "wear it down" in several ways using all the know how you have developed about this illness that can be of help, even if only partially.

Translated by Laura Monti – Milan (Italy)

The same rationale is also appropriate if you go for other options, such as Chinese medicine, homeopathy, holistic methodologies, etc.

Translated by Laura Monti – Milan (Italy)

CHAPTER III TIPS, BARRIERS, AND SOLUTIONS

As mentioned, qualitatively speaking CH is an extremely subjective disease, but also extremely varied from a quantitative point of view. What I mean is that the characteristics of CH can change enormously from an individual to the next. The intensity of the attacks can vary from bearable throughout their duration to unbearable and so strong as to induce the sufferer to seek a way out through death. In fact, CH is also known as "<u>suicide headache</u>". For these reasons it is impossible for one solution to fit all and to the same extent, but I can give you a number of tips that you can follow from time to time and see how much they can actually help you with your CH.

I wish to produce some sort of handbook as a quick and easy reference for you, providing at least one course you can follow as a way to help you pursue a transformation aimed at reducing your suffering and making you feel better.

Many of the tips you will read below may sound trivial, others very difficult. The trivial ones should not be neglected; trust them, apply them, and you will see that they make sense, they are meaningful, and don't give up on the difficult ones. Try them again and again; you will see that training, as in all other things, will make them more simple and more feasible.

Translated by Laura Monti – Milan (Italy)

HABITS

- Eat small and frequent meals and at regular times. Don't change your meal times, but keep them constant.

- Avoid sausages such as salami, particularly during the cluster phase, and all the foods that are generally contraindicated in case of headache.

- Do not eat red meat more than once a week.

- Often take probiotics, preferably homemade, such as kefiri. A web search will help you find donors of kefiri, which you can produce in a natural way at home with a little milk. Do not put kefiri in contact with aluminum or steel and avoid temperatures above 25°. Store it in the fridge in summer and out of it in winter.

- Try to eat lots of fruits and vegetables during the day. Make sure they are harvested when ripe and not submitted to artificial ripening. To this end you can look for a GAS (*Gruppo Acquisti Solidali*, or ethical purchasing group) in your region (there are many, now) and buy fruits and vegetables from them.

- Use targeted antioxidant supplements. The market offers plenty of options today, and the most effective include medicinal mushrooms such as Ganoderma, Cordiceps, Auricularia, Lions Man, etc., which should be combined with vitamin C to break their chains and promote intestinal absorption. As to vitamin C, ask your pharmacist for an extended-release formulation to ensure organic availability throughout the day.

- Try to follow a regular sleep-wake pattern, i.e. go to bed and wake up always at the same time; if you need to change your sleep-wake pattern, do it gradually, especially for awakening.

- If your energy allows it, wake up early in the morning and go for a quick walk for at least half an hour, and at night, before going to bed, do as many stretches as you can (bending on your legs) in order to promote endorphin release to ensure a good sleep.

- On holidays or weekends avoid afternoon naps. If you need to rest, use meditation or reading.

- Take effective dietary supplements, possibly prescribed *ad hoc* by a trained nutritionist.

- As far as possible, try to have a regular sexual activity.

- Avoid alcohol, smoking (if you manage), and drugs in general.

- Drink a lot of water; buy a wrist timer or use your mobile phone and set an alarm every hour to drink at least a large glass of water. Always keep a bottle of water with you to drink from.

- If the attacks are not too severe and you manage, don't take Imigran®.

- When you sense an upcoming attack, and before it becomes too severe, try to drink a RedBull® or a cup of strong coffee.

- When you are at home and you manage, at the first signs of an attack try to push it back by applying ice to your palate, hands and feet, as well as your genitals.

- At times when you often suffer from night attacks, perhaps multiple, try taking one tablet of Imigran® 100mg before bedtime and consider whether it prevents the night attack and allows you to rest. If it does, then try switching to the 50mg tablet; if it also effective, you can reduce the dose of the medication for the general benefit of your health. Improving your sleep is very beneficial in terms of reducing stress in general.

- Get an oxygen cylinder (3000 Lt) with a dispenser that delivers a flow of 7 Lt/min or faster. If it is not included in the package, call diving centers and buy one. Take dry, non-dehumidified oxygen at the first signs of an attack. To make the most of your oxygen use, when you drive or go on holiday, buy a 7Lt cylinder at diving centers and load it from time to time, even while you are on the move.

- Whenever you have the chance to stop an attack with oxygen, do it rather than use Imigran®.

- When you use oxygen to counter an attack, do so immediately as you perceive the first signs and, once the attack has subsided, continue to breathe in oxygen for another 5 minutes to prevent another attack shortly.

- If you travel by air and obtain a medical certificate from your specialist, you can take 3Lt emergency cylinders in the cabin with you.

- When an attack comes, your breathing tends to change, it becomes shorter and faster and in some cases, if the attack is severe, you tend to breathe too little. Make an effort and focus on your breathing trying to make it slower and deeper, also using your diaphragm if you manage, taking a break of a few seconds after each inhalation.

- If you happen to have nothing to stop the attack, try not to get upset – though it's very hard – as you would tend to by reaction. Try to keep calm, challenge the pain, relate with it, and plunge into meditation in pain, "relax in pain". This will not stop the attack, which will follow its course, but its duration will be shorter than if you are stiff, upset, or restless. This is, perhaps, one of the most difficult things to do, but it provides benefits in terms of reduced suffering.

- Find fifteen to thirty minutes of ME-TIME every day and learn about meditation or mindfulness, then practice them daily.

EMOTIONS, THOUGHTS, AND FEELINGS

- Don't think about cluster headache unless you're going through an attack. Don't keep thinking that you suffer from CH, that you're a loser, that you can't take it anymore, that you're disappointed, etc. Try to forget about all negative thoughts related to CH during your day (I know it's not easy, but trust me, it helps). Let these thoughts pour out and concentrate during the attack; practice until you succeed, and make sure to open a parenthesis when an attack begins and to close it when it ends. Outside of this parenthesis there should be no room for CH-related thoughts, except when you have medical checks or plan your transformation for the better with respect to CH.

- Most importantly, avoid falling into reactive depression as someone with a strong CH because of thinking continuously about your illness. It is not easy to remove thoughts from your mind, but here is a drill you can make – replace them. When the thought you need to remove arises, simply use your will to think about something else, possibly something pleasant and positive (remember the best moments in your life). By doing so you will remove that thought by simple replacement.

- Don't fight CH with your thoughts, but accept it. Accept the fact that sadly you have been hit by this illness, but luckily you have not been hit by a worse one! Accept it, accept it, don't counter it with your mind, don't deny it.

- Don't be pissed off when you talk about it to friends and co-workers that don't sympathize. Pity them, they're just ignorant because they've never tried it and are not sympathetic enough to stand by you. Forgive them, they don't do it with malice.

- During an attack, try not to stiffen in pain, but relax; surrender completely to the pain, accept it, accept that it may be a devastating illness, relax in pain. What I'm telling you may sound crazy, but it's true, if you can relax in pain, the attack is shorter. You have to do the opposite to what you would do by instinct, i.e. fidget and keep moving. People tend to get very restless during a CH attack; it is very difficult not to get restless, let alone meditate on pain, but you can do that too.

- Try not to be sad and angry. If you know how to manage your feelings, do it and avoid the anger and sadness that feed CH, but if you don't know, use meditation, which puts you in a very positive mood and gives you plenty of energy. You can learn how to do it by reading dedicated books, such as "The Orange Book, Meditation Techniques" by Osho Raynesh, or any other dedicated book that inspires and attracts you. Alternatively, there are centers that teach meditation or other channels on the internet to learn and practice it. Note that today you can use these oriental approaches, which are very useful to help change your mood for the better and slow down and reduce the flow of thoughts overloading your mind. If, for some reasons, you are against these things, turn to mindfulness, which is a sort of westernized meditation.

- Reduce the amount of thoughts you make in a day. Forget about useless thoughts: CH sufferers tend to use their mind too much, brood too much, overburden it. Slow down and think less voluntarily and consciously.

- If you are away from home and have no oxygen with you, nor Imigran® or RedBull®, in short nothing to stop an attack in the bud, then try with your mind: as you feel you are going to have an attack, forget about this feeling, don't think about it, and focus on the best moments in your life. Stick those thoughts into your mind so that they can trigger a positive emotion; this emotion, if perceived with intensity (you have to experience it, then associate it with feelings related to the five senses: sight, smell, touch, taste, and hearing), is potentially capable to push back your upcoming attack. I know these things may be quite difficult to do, but training will make them more simple and spontaneous.

MAIN BARRIERS AND HOW TO OVERCOME THEM

CH often has a progressive onset. It doesn't start as a very bad and severe disorder (though it does, in some cases), and therefore at first it tends to be underestimated, justified, and believed to be due to a period of high stress – I broke up with my partner, my mother passed away, I work too much, I sleep too little, etc.

Translated by Laura Monti – Milan (Italy)

All diseases are easier to treat if addressed upon their onset. If you have relatively short-lived night-time or day-time attacks that occur several times in a month, go straight to a good headache center and get information from authoritative sources so that you can get off to a good start with a correct diagnosis.

Then, please stop repeating to yourself such phrases as "why me, I have a terrible disease that hampers my whole life, what wrong did I do, I don't deserve this, etc.", because they sometimes generate a paranoia that doesn't help. Non-acceptance and fear arise, and they are very hard to manage.

First of all you have to acknowledge that you didn't ask for it, that you didn't do anything wrong, that it's a disease (like many others) and that, in order not to generate self-feeding psychological vicious cycles **you have to accept it as it is**, and no questions asked, full stop.

Then, when things go wrong and you can't act on it, but it keeps coming back, spoils your relax, affects your holidays, or anyway disrupts your life, you usually react with anger and gloomy or sad thoughts. There is nothing worse than anger, which feeds CH... and so does depression.

Don't give in to it, don't take a passive stance, be rational, write a headache diary and follow it, counting the time you are on and off the attacks, and you'll realize something important, namely

Translated by Laura Monti – Milan (Italy)

that, if you are about to say you always have a headache, in fact you realize it is not true as it happens with some vasomotor headaches that last whole days. In the case of CH, the attacks are just a limited part of your life.

Find a way to open a parenthesis when you have an attack and close it when it subsides, return to your ordinary life and don't think about it except to design a strategy to transform it. As to anger, physical exercise can be useful to pour it out, and meditation can help mitigate it.

A life barrier in a broad sense, CH can affect relations, both with friends and with your partner, because people tend to not understand, but their lack of understanding is not your problem, it's their problem of "ignorance". Find new friends, use the internet to get in touch with other CH sufferers. They fully understand you and know what they should and shouldn't do when you are caught in the grip of an attack. They stand by your side, they love you right away, empathy among us is something extraordinary. Maybe you will find the woman or the man of your life – I have seen it happen in OUCH Italy!

Dark thoughts and reactive depression arise when the illness becomes severe and occurs frequently.

This is another enemy that feeds CH. You must react! It's very hard but you can do it. Reactive depression is often strongest in the morning, as you wake up, and slowly fades away during the day. In some cases you will experience hyperactivity or euphoria in the evening. Particularly if you have attacks upon waking up, you have to find the strength to get up an hour earlier and go out for a run or a training session using your largest muscle masses in order to generate endorphins that wipe depression away. I know it's hard, but it's worth the effort.

Then try not to let your mind wander too much. When you realize what is going on, try to replace your bad thoughts with your best memories – this is not difficult and is something you must do! Do not withdraw, try to go out and devote to something pleasant every day to motivate your life.

Try to arrange for the implementation of the solutions you find in the book, keep a small (7Lt) oxygen cylinder (which you can buy at diving centers) in your car, as well as one or two cans of RedBull®, or caffeine concentrates for a stronger effect, and a vial of Imigran ® to take as needed.

Imigran® is a medication that is often hard to find after the months of July/August, depending on locations, and this is a big trouble for a CH sufferer that only responds to this. Talk to your doctor and buy some even if you don't need it right now, so that you will have it when needed.

Translated by Laura Monti – Milan (Italy)

CHAPTER IV MEDICATIONS

When discussing **cluster headache**, a review of the **medications** used for symptomatic and prophylactic treatment is also mandatory.

Since I am not a physician, I am only sharing my knowledge developed in my story as a CH sufferer and based on the medications I used. Everything I write also includes the notions acquired from other CH sufferers that used the same medications and participated with me in those one-to-one meetings I described above.

For cautionary reasons, you should not take and implement this information autonomously or with your GP. I recommend that you take up the information I am sharing with you and use it with your trusted neurologist to decide together on the medication-based approach that you can use to control your beast.

I am absolutely convinced that, if you establish a co-operative relation with your neurologist and demonstrate you are knowledgeable and familiar with the recommended medication, and possibly interact with him/her using the acquired knowledge and put forward your ideas and your know how (which is the story of other CH sufferers), your activity will be much more fruitful than if you just take a passive attitude.

Translated by Laura Monti – Milan (Italy)

This is the reason why I have decided to share this information, which I consider important, if not crucial. However, being cautious by nature, and for ethical reasons, I first submitted this chapter for a review to my neurologist, who also contributed by adjusting any purely medical and scientific aspects. In this respect, my wholehearted thanks go to Doctor Fabio Frediani, who is, in fact, a wonderful human being, as much as a great neurologist. Fabio, you will read this book, and I want to tell you that I learnt to love you because you deserve it, you are worthy of it.

VERAPAMIL

Verapamil (a selective calcium channel blocker acting on the heart) is the prophylactic drug par excellence used to treat cluster headache due to its good efficacy, good tolerance, and few generally sustainable side effects.

It was designed as an antihypertensive drug and intended for patients with heart disorders who have suffered heart attacks, in order to prevent potential recurrence through its vasodilating action.

The main contraindications to the intake of verapamil include heart diseases or dysfunctions, therefore, if you are naïve to the drug, you should first have an ECG (electrocardiogram) that you should submit to your prescribing neurologist. This is the practice that cautious neurologists recommend to their patients.

The maximum dose for cardiological use is 360 mg/day, while it generally ranges from 360 to 920 mg/day for cluster headache. A 240 mg/day dose can be effective for some patients that are drug-sensitive because of their own characteristics or physical weakness.

Most importantly, verapamil is usually scaled up over time until it reaches the effective dose, which is then maintained. If you are taking this medication for the very first time, you should comply with this indication for obvious cautionary reasons and assess any adverse effects. However, this intake method implies that, for the first few weeks until the effective dose is reached, you continue to suffer from the attacks that usually become less violent and more sporadic over time as the dose is scaled up, until they vanish. Moreover, this method also implies the risk of generating physical tolerance, by which the medication becomes less and less effective as the body adapts to it. In that case, the dose must be increased.

If you have already taken this medication and know what your effective dose is, I will teach you a new intake method I learned from Doctor Frediani, which very few people in Italy know and apply.

Translated by Laura Monti – Milan (Italy)

I know my effective dose is 600-720 mg/day. I take the medication right away at my effective dose as of day one and the attacks disappear within two days, so that I don't have to suffer until the effective dose is reached. By doing so, I submit my body to a mild shock *(I re-emphasize the strong impact of shocks on cluster headache)*; during the first week the side effects (bradycardia, lower blood pressure, weakness, constipation) slightly increase, but then I get used to them.

Three weeks after attacking cluster headache with verapamil, a 120mg dose reduction is performed daily or every second day, until full withdrawal. If headache returns following these reductions, the dose is immediately increased by 120mg. However, given the subjective character of each individual, you may have to scale down by less than 120mg and take the reduced dose for a longer period of time.

Bradycardia (slow heartbeat), combined with low blood pressure and subsequent weakness and increased fatigue at physical exertion, is the most common side effect of the use of verapamil. A combination with midodrine 2.5mg/ml oral drops can be effective to counter these side effects.

Another quite unpleasant side effect is constipation. Constipation is mitigated by drinking plenty of liquids, taking massive doses of bran with plenty of water or milk in the evening, or taking Laevolac® or equivalent laxatives.

Translated by Laura Monti – Milan (Italy)

Something positive about verapamil is that, unlike some other medications such as cortisone, it can be taken for extended periods of time, and is therefore also well suited for chronic CH.

Long-term intake may sometimes result into body tolerance and you have to raise the dose. If a higher dose causes unbearable side effects, the treatment should be discontinued for about a month to allow drug clearance, then the intake of verapamil can be resumed. By doing so, the previous doses remain effective in the vast majority of cases.

The intake of verapamil is indicated and effective for both episodic and chronic CH.

CORTICOSTEROIDS - CORTISONE

Cortisone is usually very effective as a prophylactic drug for cluster headache. It is the anti-inflammatory drug par excellence, and it is also a doping drug.

However, cortisone generates multiple significant and severe side effects, which make it unfit for frequent or long-term use.

The side effects of cortisone include: fluid retention, sodium retention, hypertension, heart failure, osteoporosis, loss of muscle mass, ulcers, ulcerating esophagitis, irregular menstrual cycles, excessive increase of appetite, aggressiveness, weight gain, diabetes, cataract, etc.

When taking cortisone, it is key to combine it with gastric pump inhibitors to protect the stomach and the esophagus.

The effective dose varies according to your weight and the severity of your headache, but normally you start with a high dose and then scale it down gradually. The effective daily dose is usually around 4-16mg of intramuscular Decadron® phosphate for a few days, then switching to oral Deltacortene® 25mg and 5mg scaled down by about 5mg every 3-4 days. Deltacortene® should be scaled down very gradually in order to prevent functional disruptions of the adrenal glands (an extremely severe physical reaction) that, if they occur, require the re-intake of Deltacortene® and a more gradual withdrawal. An adrenal crisis causes extreme weakness and the complete loss of physical strength. Sadly, I experienced it.

In some very tough cases of cluster headache, cortisone is used to cause a shock to the neuroendocrine system, which is often effective to stop very persistent clusters or produce a remission of chronic CH. This is called *direct drug shock* and is performed in an in-patient setting under close medical supervision.

It provides for administering 1g doses of intravenous cortisone for three or five days and then scale it down very gradually, as usual, with the use of Deltacortene®. These doses, even if taken for a limited number of days, result into a significant increase of side effects, but I stress in particular a potential increase of aggressiveness, which needs to be controlled through one's own awareness and will. However, rash overreactions to minor triggers of anger can be expected. Another important side effect is insomnia. It is therefore useful to use benzodiazepine-like medications, and/or significant doses of melatonin (even up to 10 mg) to promote sleep.

Cortisone is anyway an excellent option for some episodic CH sufferers, because it can stop the attacks for the entire duration of the cluster and prevent suffering, even if used at low doses, such as a 25mg/day tablet of Deltacortene®.

Due to the doping action of cortisone, its side effects also include some pleasant ones, such as feeling full of strength, very positive, with a hearty appetite, energetic, and in full physical shape. This is, of course, all artificial and due to the medication, but makes your life more pleasant. You may have problems upon withdrawal, though, because you get the opposite effects: you feel a little more tired, tend to sleep longer, and getting by is a little harder than before, when you were on cortisone. It is important to be aware of this, because awareness allows you to better deal with that short period, knowing that it is limited in time and will soon be over.

Translated by Laura Monti – Milan (Italy)

CARBOLITHIUM®

Carbolithium® is based on lithium salts, lithium carbonate. While it was developed as a useful medication for manic depressive psychosis or bipolar depression and as a mood stabilizer, in that it is a membrane stabilizer, it also turned out effective in the prophylactic treatment of cluster headache.

For cluster headache, however, the effective blood concentration (which should be monitored by frequent venous sampling) should be lower than required for bipolar depression.

It is an important medication to be used with caution. The main recommendation is constant monitoring of blood concentrations that, if above 1.2 mEq/l, may cause problems. It is particularly indicated in chronic CH.

A possible interaction with the endocrine system should also be considered. The thyroid function should therefore be closely monitored.

The effective dose for CH may vary among individuals, and ranges on average from 300 to 900 mg/day. However, if the higher dose is used, lithium levels should be checked at least every 15 days.

Translated by Laura Monti – Milan (Italy)

It should be noted, however, that lithium is much less effective than verapamil or cortisone.

The side effects I have experienced with lithium include emotional flattening.

ANTIEPILEPTICS

Antiepileptic drugs, which actually work as "sedatives," act as stabilizers of nerve cell membranes. For cluster headache, two have indeed been used, namely valproic acid and topiramate. Valproic acid has been used in doses of up to 2000 mg/day, with reasonable efficacy, but I never tried it personally, so I cannot report on possible side effects and alleged effectiveness. I tried topiramate, though, with significant side effects: I remember, in particular, strong annoying stings in my legs due to the direct action of the medication on the nerves. I couldn't appreciate the benefits because I still hadn't reached the effective dose, I was scaling down cortisone and also had an adrenal crisis.

It is also an appetite suppressor, and is therefore not indicated for anorexic or very thin patients.

Translated by Laura Monti – Milan (Italy)

IMIGRAN® (sumatriptan succinate 6mg subcutaneous injections and 50/100mg tablets)

Imigran® (whose active ingredient is sumatriptan succinate) interacts with the 5HT1B-D serotonergic receptors that are involved in the triggering of painful attacks, as well as in the arterial vasodilation / vasoconstriction mechanism.

Imigran® belongs to the family of triptans, introduced in the 1990s and specifically designed for the symptomatic treatment of headaches. Manufactured by Glaxo, it was then distributed and marketed by various pharmaceutical companies. Therefore the market offered multiple medications – Imigran®, Sumigrene®, Permicran®, etc. Then, for obvious reasons that I am not going to explain to avoid arguing about the socioeconomic policies of pharmaceutical companies, Glaxo remained the only company manufacturing and distributing sumatriptan.

Today new generations of triptans are available on the market for the treatment of migraine, but they are generally not effective in CH (except, in some cases, zolmitriptan - Zomig® - a second-generation triptan). Moreover, except for subcutaneous sumatriptan, which has a quick action, the other triptans are not injectable, but rather come in tablets, so that their time of action does not make them fit and effective for cluster headache.

Translated by Laura Monti – Milan (Italy)

Imigran® is, in fact, produced in several formulations: 6mg injectable vials, 10 or 20mg nasal spray, 25mg suppositories, and 50 or 100mg tablets, whose directions for use are provided below.

The Imigran® formulation normally used for cluster headache to crush an attack at the outset is the subcutaneous injection. It has a very short time of action of just a few minutes. Imigran® should be taken at the onset of an attack but, if taken during the attack, it is generally also effective. Very few people find it ineffective.

If you are naïve to Imigran®, you should be aware of its side effects: most of the times it arouses a sense of warmth that rises up to the face, often combined with a sense of constriction in the neck and chest, a sense of weakness and dereliction, and neck and head heaviness. However, while these side effects are usually intense following the injection, they are short lived, whereas the tablets' side effects are milder but more extended in time. Therefore, don't be afraid when you take it, these side effects are disturbing and scary if you are not prepared, by they are short lived. Just stretch out, try to relax, and let the medication act. You will see your attack vanish within a few minutes. They are usually stronger upon the first intake of the medication, and then subside with continued intake.

It is also important to know that in some people, including myself, that take Imigran® at the first signs of an attack, pain

Translated by Laura Monti – Milan (Italy)

tends to increase very quickly in the first minute or so. It is as if the body were countering the drug's action by opposing to it. If it happens, try to keep calm and relax in pain (we will talk about this, about how useful it is to relax in pain) and do not tense up, because otherwise it would last longer. Surrender, relax, because the medication will win and your attack will vanish within a few minutes. Sumatriptan's action is like turning off a switch – pain subsides very quickly.

The use of Imigran® is contraindicated in people with heart diseases and hypertension. Your doctor should go through your medical history before prescribing this medication. A wise doctor is usually one that asks you about this, and your GP should know you.

Imigran® tablets, on the other hand, are not generally used for cluster headache attacks, just because their time of action is much longer. However I can tell you that, if you often suffer from multiple night-time attacks and can't get a full night's sleep for some time, some CH sufferers have told me that taking one 100mg tablet of Imigran® before bedtime helps a lot in this respect. This is the only use of Imigran® tablets in cluster headache I have heard about.

Also important to know is that in many CH sufferers Imigran® is also effective at half dose, i.e. you take just 3mg of the 6mg dose contained in the vial. You may wonder how. The OUCH Italy

Translated by Laura Monti – Milan (Italy)

forum contains a video, also available on YouTube and Facebook, on how to halve an Imigran® vial. One method is described there, but I can try to explain another in a nutshell.

Remove the vial from its packaging using the self-injector and unscrewing its terminal part. Take the syringe in your hand, remove the coating paper to check the amount of liquid. Remove the refill from a ballpoint pen. Take an empty insulin syringe, then use the ballpoint pen refill to push the Imigran® injection plunger and empty half the injection into the insulin syringe. When you are done, use the insulin syringe first and then the Imigran® syringe returned into its original packaging.

Being a photosensitive drug, sumatriptan should be protected from light. I'm telling you this lest you halve the dose and do not store the unused half-vial away from light.

According to the experience of CH sufferers, frequent use of Imigran® seems to increase the attacks. This is our impression, not a certainty, and it is not proven by scientific data, but if this were the case, the rationale for halving the doses (if they are, indeed, effective) would be a smart one. You should know that the interaction between OUCH USA and the American scientific community resulted into the production of sumatriptan 4mg vials – which are, obviously, not on sale in Italy!

Translated by Laura Monti – Milan (Italy)

Imigran® is a fantastic drug for CH sufferers. It has changed my life for the better but, out of caution, in the light of the above, it should not be abused.

The medication's leaflet states that you should not have more than two injections a day, but I know dozens of people, including myself, that had more (out of obvious necessity) without having any problems. The pharmaceutical company writes that "for its own greater protection," but this often caused us procurement troubles, because physicians cannot prescribe more than one box a day for obvious professional ethics reasons.

It turns out from the experience of CH sufferers that lots of them have had more than two doses a day. An Italian professor of neurology of world-wide renown, with high competence in the field of headaches, stated in front of me that up to five vials a day should not cause heart complications. I cannot mention his name, because professional ethics would ban him saying such things as long as Glaxo does not amend the "Dosage" section in the leaflet.

Imigran® is often difficult to procure for consumers. This puts a strain on many CH sufferers in Italy, who can hardly get any supplies. When you place your order with a pharmacy, the latter usually turns to a wholesaler, and the wholesaler says the drug is out of stock. However, Glaxo has set up a toll-free number for procurement; therefore you can order Imigran® by simply calling

Translated by Laura Monti – Milan (Italy)

such toll-free number and communicate your prescription to Glaxo. Now you know! If your pharmacist doesn't, just tell him. This is clearly the current situation as I write, and I don't know whether and how things are going to change.

There is another piece of information that may be useful for chronic CH sufferers that often use Imigran® and have troubles finding it, or simply don't want to keep going to the doctor for it: a one-month stock of Imigran® can be obtained from the pharmacy of the nearest hospital. How do you achieve this? You should ask a specialized neurologist to prescribe a "therapeutic scheme" specifying your illness and your constant need for the medication. This therapeutic scheme should then be validated by your local healthcare company (if you have troubles, ask for forensic assistance). Once validated, take it to your GP, who can thus issue a prescription for as many as 30 boxes of Imigran®. With this prescription of your GP, go straight or send a fax to the pharmacy of the nearest hospital, which is obliged to procure the 30 boxes for you. Several CH sufferers, including one in the Liguria region, have already adopted this method. Considering that some health-related aspects can be addressed in different ways in each region, regions other than Liguria may have more complex or more streamlined processes. However, in case of unsurmountable difficulties, it is worth seeking forensic assistance to address bureaucratic hassles, given that the right to health is provided for by the national law, not by the regional one.

One useful thing to know if you have to travel by air and you are in a cluster is that taking Imigran® with you in the cabin requires a statement of your GP or neurologist (possibly both in Italian and in English) that you need to keep this "life-saving" medication with you, otherwise it may be confiscated at security checks.

By the way, I will tell you something funny that happened to me while travelling on a plane. I was working in Gela, Sicily, and used to fly to Milan about once a month to see my family and spend time with my girls. I think it was in 2003, and I was driving to Catania to catch an Alitalia flight to Milan.

When the aircraft's engines were started for take-off – and I was sitting next to them – I sensed an upcoming attack. Unsure whether to wait for take-off to go to the restroom and have an injection or go immediately, I decided to go immediately because the time it took from take-off to cruise level was too long for me to wait.

I decided to secretly unbuckle my belt and rush to the restroom, but the flight attendants noticed and promptly knocked on the door. I had the injection, opened the door, and fell to the ground with a suffering face. Facing this scene, the flight attendants

Translated by Laura Monti – Milan (Italy)

called the captain, who stopped the taxiing aircraft. I asked with an angry face to leave me alone and wait a few minutes for the drug to act. Meanwhile I was lying on the restroom's floor, "putting on a show". The captain came with all the flight attendants and some curious passengers to take a look.

After a few minutes, when Imigran® started to act, I got up and explained the whole story to the captain. At that point he started the "Accident" procedure and called the doctor at the Catania airport, who was supposed to assess whether I was able to continue the flight (I could hardly refrain from laughing). Meanwhile people were becoming impatient with the delay; the doctor finally arrived and asked questions, obviously in the aircraft's cabin, in front of everyone (so much for privacy!).

I explained to him that I suffered from cluster headache, that I regularly traveled by plane, that I'd had Imigran® injections before even at high altitudes (of course without anyone on the flight knowing anything about it). The next question to assess whether I could fly was, "What medications do you use?" I explained to him that I was taking verapamil and cortisone, but that unfortunately they were not very effective, they reduced the number of daily attacks, but did not completely remove my CH. Then he asked, "But why do you use cortisone?". At that point I started to feel pissed off and asked him, "Am I talking to a doctor or a newsagent? You need a training course on cluster

Translated by Laura Monti – Milan (Italy)

headache!". The doctor said, in response, "You can't fly, get off the plane."

You see, he wanted to stop me from going back home and hugging my little girls again because of his pure ignorance. Me! That's where I got mad and poured out all my anger. I got as mad as a viper and turned to the captain: "You look less stupid than this individual. Did you understand what I said and explained in front of all these people, without anyone bothering about my privacy? If you want me to get off the plane, call the police because I am not getting off and the plane won't take off. Then you will be liable for your ignorance, because I will report you to the police and tell this story to everyone."

Meanwhile, all the onlookers, who had understood, started to cheer me! Then I said to the captain: *"It is your responsibility and it is also your decision. I am aware of what I have said and I know I can fly as I always did. You should go for another doctor, because this one has no idea about cluster headache."*

Then the captain understood that things were getting rough with me, that I was not a junkie or the like, and decided to keep me on board and take off, among the passengers' cheers.

This accident is included in the official records of Alitalia and, from the care of the staff upon check-in and seat choice (once

Translated by Laura Monti – Milan (Italy)

they moved passengers, so as not to seat me close to the engines), I realized that my name had been reported.

OTHER MEDICATIONS AGAINST THE ATTACKS

Common over-the-counter medications or pain relievers, even if taken intramuscularly or intravenously, are virtually ineffective. The only one that some of the CH sufferers I was in contact with reported as helpful is **Liometacen®** (indomethacin) intramuscular or intravenous injections.

Translated by Laura Monti – Milan (Italy)

CHAPTER V DRUGS

PREAMBLE

This chapter is about the experience developed by CH sufferers with the use of certain drugs, some of which I have experienced personally while others I have never tried, but received other people's testimonies.

I have drafted a separate chapter on drugs for reasons of respect and scientific approach, but I could have included the use of drugs in the chapter dedicated to medications, because most of the medications in use for CH actually have such significant side effects that, in my opinion, they are quite similar to drugs. Moreover, certain drugs are already in use in medicine, often in countries where research is given more importance than in Italy. Italy lags far behind in this respect, even if now THC is being administered to, for example, terminal patients with cancer or multiple sclerosis. In other countries, hallucinogenic molecules are used to treat depression. While we are just about starting and going through the experimental phase, results are important and valuable in some cases. I think it is basically a matter of culture. I don't mean to be superficial but, honestly, if a drug improves my quality of life and positively counters an illness, I tend to advocate its use. I repeat, this is my personal point of view and by no means an encouragement to take drugs. I just want to convey this strong and clear message: **This is just my own testimony.**

Finally, I believe it will take years before most drugs are used for medical purposes, following reliable and strictly controlled trials, as well as minimal cultural change.

THC (DELTA-9 TETRAHYDROCANNABINOL)

Delta-9-tetrahydrocannabinol, commonly known as THC (delta-9-THC or tetrahydrocannabinol) is one of the main and best-known active ingredients of cannabis. Different types of marijuana contain variable doses of THC. THC is also found in so-called "joints", which contain a psychoactive drug obtained from marijuana.

Joints and marijuana therefore contain THC as a psychotropic substance with pain-relieving, exhilarating, anti-nausea, and appetite-stimulating properties, which can be ingested, simply smoked, or inhaled (using a vaporizer).

Nowadays, several medications containing THC are available on foreign markets, in the Vatican City or in Switzerland, as well as, increasingly, in Italy.

Translated by Laura Monti – Milan (Italy)

I will not go through the pharmacological properties of THC because this information can be easily found on the Web (always check the source!) or on PubMed, one of the most popular digital scientific libraries. Instead, I would like to inform you about the influence it may have on CH.

I would like to dwell for a moment on one important aspect, namely the administration mode of THC. While I, and others, did so at times when the medication was still unavailable (I managed to find it later), I do not recommend that you smoke pot or joints as an administration mode, for several reasons. First of all you won't be able to know how much you are taking, because buying marijuana or joints on the black market does not allow you to know what dose of the active ingredient they contain. And, by the way, you would also favor a mafia-based market. Smoking joints is definitely bad for your health, and what you buy on the black market is often a blend with other mostly unhealthy substances. These reasons are, on one hand, ethically important and, on the other, relevant from the scientific and practical point of view. If you really want to go for this option – always in strict compliance with the law – get the seeds and grow your own pot. A specialized center can also advise you on what kind of plant you should buy, and provide general information on its THC concentration.

Translated by Laura Monti – Milan (Italy)

I have never tried inhalation with a vaporizer, but it's said to be as effective and not as harmful as smoking. The ideal option is, of course, a medication, because with that you know exactly what and how much you are taking.

The first useful effect in CH is undoubtedly that it raises the pain threshold. What is the benefit of this? Raising the pain threshold slightly reduces the intensity of the attacks; therefore, in some cases, this effect allows you to cope with the attack and avoid or reduce the use of Imigran®. A chronic friend of mine, who is drug-resistant and has multiple daily attacks, mostly goes for oxygen, regularly takes THC (on prescription, and not in Italy), and reports a clear benefit. This is a prophylactic use, i.e. the medication is taken to counter an illness.

Symptomatic use is also envisaged: if you have a joint when you sense you are about to have an attack, you often abort it (this is my personal experience, shared with other CH sufferers). Since I don't want to encourage you to smoke joints, and taking the medication in tablets does not ensure that you reach the effective blood dose in due time, I recommend that you use the Sativex® sublingual spray, which I know is available in Canada and now also in Italy. It certainly has a more limited effect in time compared to tablets, but today you can easily order it online.

Translated by Laura Monti – Milan (Italy)

However, there are some aspects to consider. The use of THC for pain control also produces tolerance. This means that the dose must be scaled up over time to achieve the same effectiveness. I think this poses limits, in that it makes it suited for episodic clusters, not as much for chronic ones or, if used anyway, it should be used for a limited period of time, with withdrawal periods of at least a two or three months to allow body clearance and restore a response to sustainable doses.

On the other hand, it can be very useful in episodic cluster headache to limit the use of Imigran® (except, perhaps, in the middle of a cluster, when the attacks can become unsustainable) to avoid the risk of the beast's chronicization or, anyway, of longer cluster duration (as experienced by many CH sufferers).

I should also mention the negative feedback that I received from some CH sufferers that used it regularly, in those cases by smoking joints. They reported that, when they first had joints, their CH had improved, also in terms of fewer daily attacks, but got worse as they continued having joints. Of course, I am just reporting my own experience, and unfortunately I have no certainty and no irrefutable scientific data to share with you. This is just my personal knowledge and experience, however shared with other CH sufferers.

I can't hide from you the negative data I have collected, like the one I just mentioned. However, scientific research is closely

Translated by Laura Monti – Milan (Italy)

engaged in this regard and you can find more exhaustive scientific information by browsing the PubMed website.

Remember, though, that THC also has an influence on your mind, and may interfere with your life and your work, whether negatively or positively it depends on the individual conditions. It is still a psychotropic drug and, although many CH sufferers have tried it, my advice is to always think very carefully, and possibly also ask the opinion of a trusted doctor.

COCAINE – CODEINE

I have never tried cocaine and I don't even know of any CH sufferers that have used it for CH. Having said that, it is potentially effective as a symptomatic agent, but I think its use should be strongly discouraged, for two reasons: first, the high number of contraindications to this drug; second, using cocaine for CH implies a risk of addiction, which would pose very serious problems rather than provide benefits. In my opinion, it is not even worth trying to avoid incurring in very serious risks.

As a medication, however, there is codeine, which I have tried in the nasal spray formulation. You can obtain it with the prescription of a neurologist or a GP from "galenic pharmacies," which sell *ad hoc* preparations. The nasal spray formulation should be sprayed one to three times in the nostril ipsilateral to the attack as you sense it coming.

It is relatively effective. I mean, as I explained in my story I now have two forms of CH, one on the right, with excruciating pain, and one on the left, which is milder. Using codeine I was often able to intercept the left-side attacks, but it was ineffective for right-side ones.

I know that, a few years ago, some centers used a cocaine-based solution, but it became less and less popular over time until now it is no longer in use, probably for the above reasons.

PSILOCYBE – LSD – LSA

Let us now discuss those drugs that, despite having an important impact on people, have also been effective in producing cluster remission, to the extent that the scientific community in some countries around the world is becoming aware of CH and launching studies on it.

Such studies are currently available on PubMed, which also includes a recent Italian research carried out by Doctor Cherubino Di Lorenzo on Italian CH sufferers.

However, these experiences are reported by the Italian and American CH sufferers that used these substances and with whom I was in touch, and also include data from the Clusterbuster website, which provides information to CH sufferers on the subject.

I have no personal direct experience with LSD, I only tried psilocybe three times, as described in my story, but I received a broad variety of testimonies, both from Italy and from America, of people who enjoyed benefits and even had their life changed for the better. What is interesting about this type of drug is that it is not designed for ongoing, but rather for occasional use. I mean, once you find your effective dose for cluster remission, you just take it three times a year on average (sometimes three, sometimes two, or even one, it is very subjective).

The point is that, true, they hurt and have risks, but perhaps such an occasional use is less harmful than the ongoing use or overuse of many other medications. Also important to consider is that the required doses are lower than those used for "recreational" purposes, i.e. to get high and have hallucinations. In my experience with psilocybe, I never had hallucinations, but rather general malaise, abdominal discomfort and colics, and a more pronounced mental visualization of my thoughts, as well as a brighter color visualization. Since my experience was only limited in time, I will not mention any doses, but you can find reliable information at www.clusterbusters.com, a spin-off of OUCH USA.

Translated by Laura Monti – Milan (Italy)

It is important to know that the use of these drugs requires full clearance of medications that interact with serotonin for an extended period of time. Therefore, in order for them to be effective and not interfere with other medications, you need to be "cleared" from antidepressants, Imigran®, lithium, and even verapamil. Before you approach these drugs, you need to be well informed and wise. It should also be noted that their use is strongly discouraged for people suffering from psychosis, mental disorders, or who have a family history of this kind of disorders, because hallucinogenic molecules could reveal them. Remember that I don't want to encourage you to use these substances, I just want to inform you and tell you where you can find further details. Then it is up to you to consider your own case and assess the cost / benefit ratio of your choices. I repeat that, if your CH is under control with simple medications, such as verapamil, or you have episodic CH with long periods of respite and, perhaps, you are sensitive to cortisone, you must not consider using hallucinogenic molecules.

The action mechanism through which these drugs stop the cluster is still unclear but, in my humble opinion, it must be similar to the drug shock approach with cortisone, by which the neuroendocrine system suffers a shock downstream to which it then tends to restore its own natural biochemical balance, because everything in nature – whether micro or macro – tends towards balance.

Let's talk about psilocybe first. Psilocybe is a mushroom that grows in different parts of the world, including the Italian Alps. It contains the psychotropic alkaloids psilocin and psilocybin. There are different species of psilocybe with different concentrations of psychotropic substance. In the Italian Alps, it is easily found in September at an altitude of 1000 to 1500 meters. If you want to know what it looks like, just search "Google images" for it, you will easily find it, but be very careful, because some mushrooms that look like psilocybe may cause liver toxicity. Always beware of mushrooms. If you want to pick them up, go with an expert – DIY is not recommended. Moreover, psilocybe harvesting is illegal, and may put you in serious trouble with the law enforcement agencies. This mushroom is also found on the drugs black market, but you should not buy it there, both because you have no way to know what you are actually buying, and because you would support an illegal trade governed by the mafia. Therefore, for ethical reasons, this is not the way to go. I believe the best and safest way to go is to buy spores and grow them at home. Buying spores is not illegal and you can successfully grow them within a couple of months; you can easily find them on the internet and have them sent home.

Translated by Laura Monti – Milan (Italy)

LSD, or lysergic acid, is one of the most powerful hallucinogenic substances in the world. At minimum doses it causes hallucinations and perception alterations that may last up to eight or ten hours.

I have never used LSD because it scares me and I don't know about any other sources than the black market. I don't know any Italian CH sufferers that have used it, but only found testimonies on the internet and at an OUCH USA convention in Canada in which I participated. I personally do not recommend trying it unless you receive it in the protected environment of some experimental clinic under close medical supervision. I recommend "utmost care" with this drug: do not try or approach it out of despair, but use your brain. The best you can do is search the web for hospitals that perform trials under medical supervision and go for them!

I have no direct experience with LSA, also known as lysergamide, and I don't even know how to get or take it, but several people in OUCH Italy have more information and you can get in touch with them in the forum to learn about procurement and intake. It is 50 to 100 times milder than LSD and its effect lasts about half the time, but I understand this molecule should not be taken too lightly.

However, I received a very positive feedback in this respect from some people in Italy.

Translated by Laura Monti – Milan (Italy)

CHAPTER VI OXYGEN

Oxygen is an element of the periodic table of essential chemistry and necessary for life.

In cluster headache it is used to deal with the symptoms, i.e. to stop the attacks. Oxygen offers the best cost/benefit ratio for symptomatic treatment.

In order for oxygen to be most effective, it must be taken immediately, at the first signs of the attack. If you have shadows before the attacks or perceive alterations (as it happens in many cases) suggesting that an attack is coming, that is the best time to start taking it.

If the attack is already under way, oxygen is often still effective to stop it, but sometimes, in some people, it doesn't work.

In most cases oxygen is usually effective, except in some individuals that suffer from very strong attacks and particularly severe cluster headache.

In order for oxygen to display its full potential, you should know how to properly take it. First of all the oxygen flow should be high, usually between 7 and 15 Lt./min. Oxygen intake should be performed via a non-rebreathing mask, fitted with a balloon.

Translated by Laura Monti – Milan (Italy)

They are not difficult to find today, particularly on the internet, but if you are in trouble just ask the OUCH Italy forum.

In order to know what is the right flow for you, always start with the maximum flow, then gradually reduce it at each attack until you notice it becomes ineffective.

Also in view of achieving maximum effectiveness in stopping an attack via oxygen breathing, note that oxygen should not be humidified. If the delivery system mounted on the cylinder is fitted with a bubbler, if possible remove it, otherwise do not fill it with water (which is the reason for its presence).

In most people, oxygen is effective at first, i.e. it stops the attack, but then the attack recurs within a short time, as if it had not been completely sedated. In order to avoid this unpleasant inconvenience, continue to take oxygen for another five minutes after the attack has subsided, possibly at a lower dose.

When taking oxygen, attacks usually subside within 5-10 minutes, but it can also take longer in more difficult cases.

Oxygen intake at the above doses can easily cause dizziness. While oxygen is said to be harmless and not bad for one's health, it is in fact the oxidant par excellence, and cell oxidation is the main cause for aging and for a number of disorders. In fact, studies on longevity are aimed at creating specific antioxidants acting at different oxygen levels. This is to warn you that you

Translated by Laura Monti – Milan (Italy)

should not fall asleep with your mask on, nor take oxygen for extended periods of time: if you experience no benefit within 15-20 minutes, you should stop delivery.

Pharmacies usually provide 3000Lt. oxygen gas cylinders. They are quite large, you can keep them at home but they make the use of oxygen difficult and impractical at work or when you're out. However, here are some solutions to this.

Diving equipment stores sell 7Lt. cylinders that provide 1540 Lt. at a 220 kPa pressurization. This type of cylinder is quite small, but offers reasonable convenience. You can keep it in your car or take it on holiday with you, and safely recharge it at diving centers. Smaller 3Lt. cylinders are also available, but they are definitely less convenient.

In the past, most CH sufferers found it hard to obtain the oxygen prescribed by their GP, in that it was not described as a "medication" (if I can call it that) in the treatment protocols for cluster headache. Most of the times the prescription of a specialized neurologist was required and, in some cases, it was even hard to get a neurologist to recommend and prescribe it.

In the light of the above, several no-profit organizations started to advocate the inclusion of oxygen into protocols for CH. A petition was also drafted on the subject, which many CH sufferers, their families, and other people signed.

Translated by Laura Monti – Milan (Italy)

Things have changed **since the AIFA resolution including oxygen in the lists of medications for consolidated use in the treatment of Cluster Headache attacks, in accordance with Law 648/96 (prot.1153/15 of 14.11.2015), was published in Official Journal No. 12 of 16.01.2016:** now we CH sufferers can demand that oxygen be prescribed to us.

Oxygen is not a gas to be taken lightly, you should get familiar with it and learn to manage it. Oxygen is one of the three elements of the fire triangle, i.e. a fire feeder, the combustion agent required to "give life" to fire, together with the fuel and the temperature required for ignition. Do not keep 220 kPa pressurized cylinders too close to heat sources.

Most importantly, you should shut the main valve of the cylinder after use.

Currently available cylinders are usually fitted with a protection device around the valve, but some may not have it. In this case, always store the cylinder safely, ensuring it doesn't fall over (sometimes they are supplied with a fall-arrest device, or you can buy such device to prevent falls). This is very important because the vulnerable point of the cylinder is located at the supply valve connection. If this point is hit and broken upon falling, the 220 kPa pressurization would cause the cylinder to start like a rocket and destroy everything around.

Translated by Laura Monti – Milan (Italy)

According to the law, cylinders should be tested every 5 years for safety. A marking of the latest test is stamped on the nosepiece of the cylinder, which is the top colored part.

If the above information is not enough for you, you can refer to the OUCH forum, or to Al.Ce. Fondazione Cirna onlus.

It is also important to know that back in the 1990s oxygen was administered in the hyperbaric chamber for cluster headache prophylaxis. In some cases it was effective and made the attack subside. In a hyperbaric chamber, you take oxygen at a 1.5 bar pressure, which raises the partial pressure of oxygen in your blood.

However, going to a hyperbaric chamber may cause logistic challenges and I notice that (whether for economic or other reasons) it is hardly ever prescribed by neurologists as a method for CH prophylaxis. However, it is a less invasive, albeit not very practical option compared to medication intake, and thus worth a try.

Translated by Laura Monti – Milan (Italy)

CHAPTER VII THE FIRST ALLY, VERY OFTEN DISREGARDED - WATER

I trust you will forgive me if some of the things I mention sound obvious, but **obvious things** tend to be taken for granted and **not given due consideration**. The solutions to serious problems are often sought in large-scale and complex approaches, while they are within reach in small things that border on obviousness.

As you will have by now understood, I am not providing you the solution to recover from CH, **but only to suffer less and improve your quality of life.**

I realized that not everyone is aware of the obvious uses of water, some ignore them and, when they start to adopt them, they feel better! This is why I think it is useful and appropriate to address this topic, which is very simple and within everyone's reach.

Air, water, and food for the "Human Machine" are the three necessary elements for survival and are listed in order of time-based need. This means that, if you give air with less than 19% of oxygen to your body, you will die within a few minutes. If you give it no water, you will die within a few days (three to five). If you give it no food, you will die within a few months.

Translated by Laura Monti – Milan (Italy)

Let us now talk about water. The human body is made up of 75/80% water. Most electrolysis processes occur if there is good hydration; the blood can circulate correctly and clotting is avoided only if the body is well hydrated. The intestine functions correctly and does not tend to harden if the body is well hydrated. In short, I am not going to list all the reasons to ensure good body hydration, because they alone could be the subject of an entire book, but **it is important to know that a lack/shortage of water may hamper proper body functioning.** If you have malfunctions or weaknesses, whether of the stomach, the intestine, the joints, or the **head**, inadequate water intake tends to make them worse.

Scientific studies have already shown that headache sufferers in general (including those with CH, as well as other forms of headache) tend to be under-hydrated.

Now try to think for a moment whether you also belong to this group of people: if you don't drink at least two liters of water per day in winter and three in summer, **you might be one of the lucky ones that see their CH improve by only increasing their daily water consumption.**

I will go back for a moment to why. What CH exactly is is still unknown from the scientific point of view, but from the holistic point of view it may be seen as originating from a malfunction of the neuroendocrine system, which goes haywire and generates

Translated by Laura Monti – Milan (Italy)

too many impulses that reach the cortex and, for whatever reason, trigger a CH attack.

If your neuroendocrine system, your "body machine", is weak in this respect and you hamper its operation (in many ways, not just with a water deficit), it will display this weakness more often. It is easier to understand than to describe! Our neuroendocrine system is particularly sensitive to stressors of whatever nature, whether induced by feelings, overexercise, environmental factors (sudden temperature drops, sudden thunderstorms), etc. Have you ever noticed the effects of sudden climate changes on your CH? They are due to the fact that your system is not able to react adequately to the environmental stressor to which it is exposed.

However it is often a matter of awareness: if you are not aware of these and continue with your poor drinking habits, this will continue to cause you troubles; **if, instead, you become aware and, indeed, you strive to drink more and better**, you will also draw benefits in terms of lower number of attacks or reduced pain intensity.

I will try to explain what I mean by drinking more and better. More is easy: you increase your average water consumption to about three liters per day and some more in summer, because of more intense dispersion with transpiration.

Translated by Laura Monti – Milan (Italy)

Better means that you should not wait until you feel thirsty to drink, because when you feel thirsty **your body is already suffering a water deficit and therefore reacts by giving you signals that you need water** (the human body, and nature, are smarter than you think), so try to drink before that happens, try not to make your body suffer from water shortage. It's like a car, you need water to cool down the engine, otherwise it overheats and fails. Water should never fall below the minimum level, or the red warning light on the dashboard starts to flash. **Our thirst is equivalent to the red warning light that flashes on your car's dashboard whenever the cooling water drops below the minimum level.**

First of all, try to get used to drinking a large glass of water every hour. If you tend to forget, set an acoustic countdown every hour (as I do to remember taking my pills at noon, which I tend to forget), then get into the habit of always taking a one-pint bottle of water with you that you can refill with drinking water every time it's empty.

It should be known and understood that sometimes the attacks arise from a shortage of water in the body, due to the above reasons, and that changing habits (learning to drink at least three liters of water a day) is not always easy. Once you know this rule for drinking, **you have to apply it – knowing is not enough, you**

Translated by Laura Monti – Milan (Italy)

have to act (this applies to everything in life: **A small deed is worth more than broad knowledge**).

If the upcoming attack is caused by a reaction of your "system" to the water shortage stressor, a quick intake (however swallowing slowly) of a pint of fresh water often stops it, but it is crucial that you do so immediately, that you begin to drink at the first signs of the attack, rather than wait until the attack has reached its peak.

Look at yourself as if you were an external observer and consider whether you drink too little or the right way. If you drink too little, strive to drink more, drink two or three liters of water throughout the day. Then, when you feel that an attack is coming (we know there are warning signs: some call them shadows, others experience them as general discomfort or intolerance to everything around; anyway, on average we sense an upcoming attack), drink a pint of water quickly.

If what I'm saying – addressing such a severe illness as CH by drinking plain water – sounds like nonsense, I advise you not to think about it, not to dwell too much upon it, but to try, to **take action**. All in all, you have nothing to lose, **but if it works for you, you've got an extra weapon to "wear down" the beast.**

Translated by Laura Monti – Milan (Italy)

CHAPTER VIII FOOD AND FOOD SUPPLEMENTS

"Wearing down CH" means being able to interact positively with all the aspects connected with and affecting it that lead to its improvement, albeit partial.

The effort to put our "Human Body Machine" in the best working conditions also involves nutrition and food supplementing.

As far as nutrition is concerned, some forms of migraine are triggered by certain foods, such as chocolate, sausages, red wine, cheese, etc. This is not the case for cluster headache, though. In my one-to-one work described in the introduction and in the investigations carried out by OUCH Italy in cooperation with a highly qualified professor, **two uncommon, but peculiar aspects were observed in some CH sufferers.**

In some, the crises were triggered also after eating some foods (such as chocolate or sausages), while in others the attacks improved significantly after eliminating some foods that caused intolerance. CH IS NOT A FOOD-RELATED MIGRAINE (I wrote it in block letters to prevent misunderstandings), nor a tension-type headache, but since it still belongs to the class of cephalalgias, links may exist with other types of headache/migraine.

Translated by Laura Monti – Milan (Italy)

Therefore, if a CH sufferer is under stress for some reason, such stress may trigger an attack; similarly if a CH sufferer is intolerant to tomatoes, consuming tomatoes may trigger the attack, probably because of the introduction of an additional stressor into a body that is susceptible to stressors.

Based on my observations that span over twenty years of analysis of my own and other peoples' CH, I can thus claim that the following two approaches may help: the first is to have a food intolerance test at a highly qualified center to see whether you are intolerant to any foods and, if so, eliminate them from your diet and observe any influence on your CH; the second is to take note of what you eat in a diary to see whether there are any foods that trigger your attacks, in which case you eliminate them.

A common trait in almost all CH wear-down activities is stressors. **If you eat a food you're intolerant to, you'll put your body under stress!**

For CH sufferers, stress is a common trait that influences their illness.

Food supplementing is useful for two reasons: on one hand, CH sufferers tend to overconsume certain compounds (salts and vitamins) and, on the other, current dietary habits in

Translated by Laura Monti – Milan (Italy)

industrialized countries often include industrial foods processed through supply chains. Here is an example of this.

Today, the orange (or any other fruit) you buy at the supermarket was not picked from the tree when ripe, having developed all its compounds (primarily vitamin C), but was picked unripe and ripened using artificial methods. **This type of ripening impoverishes the fruit,** and the same is true for most produce (unless you have your own countryside orchard or your own garden).

While it is certainly healthier to adopt a diet as balanced and genuine as possible, this is difficult in present times and you can therefore support your diet with food supplements.

The long-term suffering caused by CH, as well as by other forms of headache and migraine, results into severe oxidative stress and into the overconsumption of certain substances in the body.

In cluster headache sufferers it is important to supplement such substances as vitamins B or magnesium, because they help improve the body's functioning and reaction to stressors.

A vitamin-based therapy (if we want to call it that way, even if it is not really a therapy) is usually very long and should be continued for months, yet it can be effective because it helps improve the functioning of our body machine through the intake of the salts and vitamins it needs, which reduces its stress.

Translated by Laura Monti – Milan (Italy)

However, a targeted vitamin and salt-based therapy requires **relying on professional advice, possibly of a nutritionist, or even your GP.**

I say this because if you take vitamins without having the proper knowledge, you can make two basic errors: the first is they are not effective and are wasted. This is the case, for example, of vitamin C: if you take even as much as one whole gram of vitamin C (which is quite a high dose), your body absorbs the dose it needs at that moment (e.g. a few milligrams) as soon as it receives it and eliminates the rest. You may be sure you took one gram, but in fact you almost eliminated it all because your body took what it needed and nothing more. In this case, to make up for this inconvenience, you need to take vitamin C-Tard®, vitamin C that is gradually released so that the amount needed over 12 hours is always available to the body.

The second mistake, which is much more serious, is that if you take too much vitamin of a certain type, for example group B vitamins or vitamin D, you may cause what is known in medicine as hypervitaminosis, which causes problems of a varying nature depending on the vitamin you have overconsumed.

For this reason, not being a nutritionist, I don't want to talk about doses because vitamins and salts depend on a **daily dose that, however, a nutritionist can adjust according to individual subjectivity.** I will now give you **some general information, but I**

urge you not to follow strictly what you read, but to learn a lesson and then turn to a skilled nutritionist.

The supplements I used and suggest include:

- Vitamins B - B2, B6, B12, etc.
- Vitamin C
- Vitamin A
- Vitamin D
- Tryptophan
- Magnesium
- Potassium
- Vitamin E
- Coenzyme Q10
- Zeolite
- L-Tryptophan
- Medicinal mushrooms such as Ganoderma, Lion's man, and Cordiceps

Something I wish to mention, although I have not experienced, is the use of vitamin D and, if I understand correctly, of vitamin D3. Based on American experiences, it seems the targeted use of

Translated by Laura Monti – Milan (Italy)

vitamin D3 may even stop the attacks. I never met or interacted with the Americans that used it, but I found this information in OUCH Italy, where a bunch of people who don't take any medications except Imigran® said they tried vitamin D3 in America and managed to stop the attacks. Back to Italy, they continued to take this supplement and the benefit persisted. You can find this information at https://goo.gl/zWqfKB.

However, be careful and monitor the intake dose with blood tests, because hypervitaminosis from vitamin D is very harmful to the body. I urge you to gather abundant information through OUCH Italy and to have dedicated supplementation under medical supervision.

Food supplements also include probiotics that feed the intestinal flora, and deserve a dedicated discussion.

The new frontiers of (non-allopathic) medicine see the intestine as a second brain, with a separate intelligence that has a significant influence on brain biochemistry and on the immune system.

It seems intestinal malfunctions can lead to biochemical alterations, and that constipation and retention of feces can increase body intoxication!

Have you ever noticed that, at the hardest CH times, you get diarrhea (serotoninergic nexus)? How comes the use of

Translated by Laura Monti – Milan (Italy)

verapamil, which stops the cluster, makes you constipated? Why does a severe shock cause evacuation (adrenergic nexus)? The reasons are still largely unknown, but meanwhile **let's take care!**

Good intestinal functioning is very important, as currently shown by specific studies!

Probiotic supplements to keep the intestine in good shape are definitely useful to ensure the proper functioning of our brain biochemistry. Few medical schools teach this, because unfortunately most tend to stick to old notions, but perhaps we should start talking about it.

Excellent supplementing with fresh and varied live cultures (better than the probiotics sold in pharmacies) can be obtained with Kefiri supplemented with milk for fermentation. Live probiotic kefiri can be found free of charge on the internet; users generally give the reproduced probiotics away for free. By doing so, first you incur in no expense (except for the little amount of milk you use for fermentation), and second, the strains produced by the Kefiri are even more abundant than those you find as probiotics in pharmacies.

The next subject is cell oxidation. On one hand, oxidative metabolism is a source of energy but, on the other, it produces free radicals that damage cell membranes and other biological structures (lipids, proteins, DNA, etc.).

Translated by Laura Monti – Milan (Italy)

Just consider that the formation of free radicals is the basis for the onset of many illnesses, as well as for aging.

Free radicals are particles with unpaired free electrons that make them unstable, short-lived, and highly reactive.

Consider that antioxidants and melatonin are at the basis of scientific studies on longevity!

An overproduction of free radicals occurs in CH sufferers, and therefore antioxidant supplements are very useful to improve the proper functioning of our "body machine."

It is important to know that antioxidants come in different types of a varying nature (e.g. vitamins, such as vitamin C) and that they are contained in food, particularly in fruits and vegetables if harvested when ripe.

The above-described food marketing rationale reduces the antioxidant power of food. This is to remind that there is nothing better than a good and proper diet that, however, is still not always enough, and that's where food supplements come into play.

I tried some good antioxidants, such as fermented papaya. It is sold in pharmacies at fairly high prices, but it is very good (be sure to go for a high-quality product from a reliable pharmaceutical company, not a by-product or one on sale in supermarkets).

Translated by Laura Monti – Milan (Italy)

The most powerful antioxidant I have found, which contains a 12000 orac value of antioxidant power, is called DAILY Fusion®, but it is no longer available.

Another very effective antioxidant is Zeolite, which is alleged to reduce oxidation by 18%, but in this case I suggest that you do your own search on the web and assess website reliability and product quality. You can also consider supplementing your diet with turmeric that, if associated with black pepper, also contributes to promote neuron proliferation, or with ginger.

Other truly excellent antioxidants include medicinal mushrooms, such as Ganoderma or Reishi, Cordiceps, Lions man and others. Ten species are approved in Italy. Medicinal mushrooms contain multiple compounds, in addition to antioxidants, and are also useful to boost the immune system and nourish the intestinal bacterial flora, detoxify, etc. Mycotherapy is a branch of phytotherapy that has been tested for over 4000 years in the East and is widely used today in Europe and America. The EC set up a scientific research committee for mycotherapy, which also boasts anti-cancer potentials (see Directives 2001/83/EC and 2004/24/EC, http://www.ema.europa.eu/). In Italy it is still almost unknown.

The above are just hints based on the products I use, but it is always best to refer to a skilled nutritionist capable to design a dedicated supplementing scheme.

Translated by Laura Monti – Milan (Italy)

Another important supplement is melatonin.

Melatonin is produced in the brain in the evening around bedtime and is a conversion, a *transformation of serotonin*.

CH sufferers normally have troubles falling asleep, they often fear sleeping, in that the attacks often come at night, during the REM phase. Serotonin levels fluctuate and CH sufferers tend to worry. Worrying while trying to go to sleep hampers the whole process.

CH sufferers often have a disrupted sleep-wake cycle, which is influenced by the onset of the attacks. Have you ever noticed that, if on some days you stay longer in bed, you have an attack? Have you ever noticed that changes in your sleep-wake cycle bring about changes in the time of your attacks? (They usually occur at fixed times, which can vary if the sleep/wake cycle is disrupted).

In view of supporting these changes, many CH sufferers benefit from melatonin supplementing (albeit just in terms of improved sleep quality).

While the dose that is normally prescribed for jet-lag disorders is 1 to 3mg, the dose for CH sufferers can be as high as 9-10 mg. This should help you go to sleep earlier and enjoy a more restful sleep. In more severe cases you can raise the dose to 20-30mg.

Melatonin should be taken before bedtime.

Translated by Laura Monti – Milan (Italy)

Since the discovery of all its benefits (first and foremost its anti-aging action), melatonin has been marketed by dozens of manufacturers.

Melatonin is currently sold in 1mg doses, whereas the 3 and 5mg doses have been withdrawn from the market. It is therefore useful to buy liquid melatonin, which you can dose at will.

I strongly advise that you do not buy melatonin at the supermarket, even if is cheaper, but rather choose a certified product sold in pharmacies and manufactured by some pharmaceutical company, so as not to risk failing in your attempts because of poor quality.

To sum it up, I wish to point out that, while CH has nothing to do with headaches due to food intake or food intolerance, it turned out useful in some cases to monitor the diet to assess whether the attacks were associated with the intake of specific foods and, in others, eliminating foods that caused intolerance dramatically improved the attacks.

The idea is to minimize the stressors to which our body is exposed.

For the purpose of ensuring that our body is in the best working conditions, it is useful to arrange for a targeted intake of certain supplements, including vitamins, minerals, melatonin, and antioxidants.

Translated by Laura Monti – Milan (Italy)

THE KETOGENIC DIET

Last but not least, I want you to know that I have heard of some CH sufferers who described improvements of their CH on Facebook using the **ketogenic diet**. I had no idea what this diet was ("keto" what?), and tried to get some useful information and insights. This is how I met Doctor Cherubino Di Lorenzo, a specialist in this field and the first researcher to apply the ketogenic diet to CH sufferers with interesting results. It is an option that deserves a try, though being quite a challenge. Being completely new to it, I will just share with you the limited information I have, and invite you to search for more details and, possibly, have a try, supported by specialists in this specific field.

Tests are still under way and Doctor Di Lorenzo is in touch with the OUCH. He has also created a private group on Facebook to address this topic and provide his testimonies. The group is called "Ketogenesis."

Ketogenesis is a physiological phenomenon that occurs in all mammals in case of prolonged fasting or low carbohydrate intake. A diet is called ketogenic when it is able to trigger the formation of ketone bodies, i.e. ketogenesis. For over a century the ketogenic diet (of which several types exist) has been used to treat patients with drug-resistant epilepsy or patients that were

Translated by Laura Monti – Milan (Italy)

unable to take medications, as well as for slimming. Since the 1920s, the efficacy of ketogenesis has often been observed in migraine and other neurological disorders.

Through the information I collected, as well as reading interviews with Doctor Di Lorenzo (E-bulletin, CIRNA Fondazione Onlus, No. 80 May 2012), I found that, ever since the age of Hippocrates, applying this diet brought about an improvement in seizures.

The diet was used by chance for the prophylaxis of migraine in 1928, when Doctor Charles Francis Schnabel of the Kansas City Rockhurst College presented a study with very promising results. The study was intended to demonstrate the usefulness of wheatgrass as a food supplement in poor diets. In fact, wheatgrass is rich in proteins, vitamins, and minerals and an unexpected therapeutic effect of this food was also observed in migraine.

Ketone bodies are the product of the transformation of fat deposits into an energy substrate to help survive through prolonged fasting.

With its excellent ability to "burn" ketone bodies, the human brain extracts a large amount of energy, which is more noble.

In fact, if I understood correctly, the energy produced by the "fat fuel" is nobler than that produced by the "carbohydrate fuel".

This diet is based on a very low intake of carbohydrates.

Translated by Laura Monti – Milan (Italy)

An article in *Focus* (which, I think, is a reliable scientific magazine) of March 2017 claimed: "*Here is the diet against migraine. If you suffer from migraine, you can prevent the attacks by eating more fat and less carbohydrates. This was the finding of a group of researchers at the University of Rome La Sapienza, led by Cherubino di Lorenzo, which reintroduced a diet created over 100 years ago to treat childhood epilepsy. This diet mimics fasting, thus causing the body to use the ingested fats to produce specific chemical compounds, known as "ketone bodies." A ketone body contains more energy than glucose (which derives from carbohydrates). Thus neurons can better make up for the brain energy deficit that triggers migraine. In a trial performed on a sample of 100 women, the number of days with migraine in a month fell from 5.1 to 0.9. DV*"

Later I had the opportunity to read some testimonies of both migraineurs and CH sufferers, who drew significant benefits from this diet, but beware of a very important aspect: this type of diet cannot be a do-it-yourself option; you must seek the advice of an expert and, if you are a CH sufferer and/or are acquainted with migraineurs, you should join the research group created by Doctor Di Lorenzo to assess whether it can be beneficial for you. I have also heard it is not easy at first, because it overturns your dietary habits and you need to arrange carefully for it.

Translated by Laura Monti – Milan (Italy)

CHAPTER IX THE HOLISTIC VISION

INTRODUCTION

The concept of "holistic vision" should now be applied to your illness. What is it about? What does it mean...? It is **the biological theory by which the body should be considered in its entirety and wholeness, rather than as a sum of parts.**

For centuries, the East and the West have been separated by different visions of reality and of life. In the West, the hyper-development of the intellectual dimension has resulted into the undisputed benefit of scientific and technological progress, however combined with an impoverishment of our existence and the loss of a "holistic" vision of life. All civilizations and traditions have always shared a sacred and unitary vision of existence. Some, like the eastern ones, partly maintain their characteristics, while others, like the western ones, forgot about their roots.

An important consequence for the West was the separation between the mind and body, caused by a hyper-development of rational logics and, therefore, a separation between the two fundamental wisdoms: the intellectual and abstract one and the "holistic", unitary one, concerned with the body and mind taken

Translated by Laura Monti – Milan (Italy)

together, direct and straightforward, which means closely participating with all one's being.

The above is easy to understand but, to give you a clearer idea of what I mean by dealing with CH according to a "holistic vision," I will give you some practical examples. If your liver is enlarged or hurts, you go to a specialized hepatologist, who prescribes clinical tests and ultrasound scans to check the conditions of your liver, as well as medications to treat the symptoms or improve your test results. However, liver disorders can also originate from a wrong approach to life, including being furious, always angry, too perfectionist, and seeing wrong in other people, which is often at the origin of anger. In this case, whatever medications you take (according to the western vision), you will never solve the problem, i.e. its cause, and your illness can only get worse, not least because the liver, as the purifier of the body, will also have to filter out the medications you take. In this *"specific reported case," I think the western vision is a loser.*

Another example is a sore stomach and esophagus, perhaps due to reflux esophagitis that, in western medicine, is studied specifically on the concerned organs. However, it can be a result of too much stress in the broadest sense and therefore cannot be solved using proton pump inhibitors or performing stomach PH-metry. The disorder persists and may develop into a carcinoma of the esophagus, an organ that is not designed to resist to the acidity of gastric juices. The solution is stress mitigation and constant meditation to relax the cardias, i.e. the valve that separates the esophagus from the stomach, and ensure its proper functioning.

Other examples include headache in the broadest sense, including CH, or colitis, pain-related muscular contractions, sometimes generating vertebral subluxations, etc.

Both visions (the eastern and the western one) have limits but, if integrated, their outcome can produce exponential improvements in the medical field.

Luckily today, more and more health operators (those with a slightly more futurist vision) are already working along this line.

PRIMARY HEADACHE

Primary headache is a headache that has no physical triggers. If a headache is due to a cyst that developed in your brain, a carotid occlusion, cancer, or other similar organic causes, it is called secondary headache. On the other hand CH, like migraine and many other forms of headache, is defined as primary because it has no specific cause.

Translated by Laura Monti – Milan (Italy)

Despite their complexity, nature and our body have a superior intelligence. As we look at our brain, which is still largely unknown, such superior intelligence can be observed. When I speak of this form of intelligence I do not refer to our own intelligence, which resides in the frontal lobe, but rather to a superior intelligence that sees the brain as an organ in its entirety. If "sick," our brain (including emotions and spirit) is able to trigger inner diseases, as well as organic ones but, if properly managed, it is also able to heal existing diseases or diseases that it triggered in the first place: its intelligence and skills are truly first-rate!

Primary headache, whatever its etiology, has a common trait, pain in the head, that is, your head simply aches.

I try to make it simple because the solutions to big problems are most often found in simple things. They may be just there in front of you, but you don't see them because you are blinded by your compulsive search for difficult solutions, and your brain is in a cloud.

We talked about pain, but **what is pain and what is it meant to tell us?** Pain is your ally for survival! To put it simply, imagine you are a young child who is learning life, and you face fire. You had never seen fire before and you find it very attractive. You are alone, no adult is there to explain that you must not touch it, nor to protect or direct you. Being attracted by it, you walk closer

Translated by Laura Monti – Milan (Italy)

and instinctively try to touch it, perhaps slowly, cautiously, but you do. As you approach it, your hand makes you feel pain and, because of such pain, you take it back and thus avoid being burnt. This is the intelligence I told you about – the natural intelligence of our body.

What did pain do in this particular case? It protected you, it prevented you from getting burnt and taught you that something as beautiful as fire should just be looked at, but not touched! **Pain always plays the same function: protect you and teach you something!**

We said that headache is pain in the head. What does it want to protect us from? What does it want to teach us? The brain is comparable to a muscle and you have to train it for use! What happens if you go for a long race without training? The next day at the least you have pain in your thighs and calves, because of lactic acid, which tells you that you have to address such efforts more gradually, you have to train slowly and increase your effort gradually. Couldn't it be the same for your head, which houses your brain? Couldn't it be that, if we use our brain too much, we get a headache? I leave the answer to you because I think I already have my own answer, though I can't be sure!

I really encourage you to think about these things, because they make a lot of sense, and can even provide helpful solutions for you!

Translated by Laura Monti – Milan (Italy)

If headache is pain in the head, according to a holistic vision it is up to us first, also with the help of specialists, to understand what it wants to protect us from and what it wants to teach us!

WHAT THE BEAST MEANS TO TELL US

Some background information before talking about cluster headache. There is no "ultimate remedy" for cluster headache, no one-size-fits-all. A remedy can work for some but not for others, but this doesn't mean it is not effective as such. CH should be approached in multiple and different respects in order to know, understand, and tame it, but always with a "holistic-vision-of-the-problem" approach integrated with western medical wisdom.

CH is a disorder with countless different facets, which change from an individual to the next, and this is why the same prognosis can hardly fit different people. An analysis to identify possible winning strategies should be designed and performed on each individual, in search of the best approaches to "wear it down" based on the knowledge you have from time to time of your CH, in order to counter it and change its course. I also call CH *mal de vivre*, a subjective illness, because it hints to a deep imbalance towards life. This imbalance can then be on a million

Translated by Laura Monti – Milan (Italy)

different levels from person to person, each in different spheres and profiles.

For this reason, *you* are the best doctor for your CH. You should not take a passive attitude, but rather a proactive one, making sure that you don't get the solution from the professional operators you seek advice from, but rather create alliances with them to help you understand it according to a well-defined "holistic vision", being aware that the problem is not limited to simple vasodilation that produces trigeminal inflammation that generates pain. Hypothalamic hyperactivity during an attack seems to be demonstrated, but in my opinion – as I wrote in the OUCH forum years ago – the problem goes even deeper, is "rooted in the amygdalae"!

Let us have a closer look. CH in general causes a sharp pain that may appear several times a day and stops you from doing anything you are doing. It blocks you, nothing else exists and, during the acute phase, it causes 100% disability and keeps you away from anything else. It may be trying to draw your attention away from a serious problem, to stop and prevent you from doing something stressful; it may even want to stop you from thinking and using your brain (during an acute attack, mere thinking made my pain even stronger). It may be the intelligence of your body sending a really important message that you cannot

Translated by Laura Monti – Milan (Italy)

afford to ignore, or it comes back and doesn't let you live as you are doing.

In fact, it changes your life when it's bad, it doesn't let you drink alcohol, it doesn't let you enjoy a quiet night out with your friends, it makes you feel anxious about simply going out for shopping without your vials of Imgran® with you, there is nothing it lets you do (during the attacks). In short, it tells you, "You must look at me and listen to me!"

Of course I am not sure about what I say, it just popped up in my mind and I want to share it with you to take you – if you are not already there – to a visual level that has a higher energy frequency, and can offer an added value to help you **transform your beast**. My purpose – as I wrote at the beginning of this book – is to help you suffer less. *If I could, you certainly can!* I didn't succeed within a few months, it took years of suffering, but perhaps this book can help reduce the time you need to tame your own beast. This is something I wish you with all my heart.

When I speak about the holistic concept, I do not intend to demonize western medicine that, with its approach, gave us so much for many illnesses, but I rather want to convey a pressing need to integrate the eastern and western medical wisdom (something made possible by globalization). Some people are already doing so.

Translated by Laura Monti – Milan (Italy)

For example, western medicine uses statistics to give us information that can also be used in the holistic approach. Statistics say that CH sufferers tend (and I stress "tend to," because I have known cases that were not) to be overactive, ultra-busy people, employers or mobbed and bullied employees overwhelmed with responsibilities. This alone is quite telling: usually a CH sufferer is not a quiet person, but a brooding and stressed one! This information provides food for thought: look at yourself, does it mean you? If it does, you already have a plan to work on to change. I don't mean that, if you are an entrepreneur, you should become an employee, but that maybe ten minutes in the morning and ten minutes in the evening for meditation can be of great help to slow down your mind and dissolve some of your stress. I chose this example, but there could be hundreds. What matters is that you work on yourself!

<u>In my review, I believe that CH originates from a post-traumatic stress you are not over!</u> That CH has to do with stress is something I'm sure of. **Stress is the hypothalamic reaction to a change;** such change is not only for the worse, but also for the better (in fact, any change requires adaptation), but it still causes stress. Think about it: did you ever happen to experience severe stress at work, then go on vacation, suddenly relax, and your CH gets worse? It happens to me and to many other CH sufferers with whom I spoke. I think it's because "hypothalamic reactivity" finds it difficult to counter stressful events of any kind and type!

UNDERSTANDING AND INFLUENCING THE BEAST

Observation is the magic word, but even more magic is observing yourself from the outside. Write down or record everything you observe about yourself, lest you forget. While it is not too difficult to observe what you do during the day, how stressed you are, if you brood too much, etc., it is more difficult to observe yourself as an onlooker.

What do I mean?

Did you ever happen to be a good advisor, to find the solution to a problem of your friend's but be unable to find the solution to your own problem? I went through that very often, and I wish to share my experience with you, but it's something many other people experience as well. The difference is that when dealing with your friend's problem you are not fogged or distorted by his or her emotions, conditionings, or biases, but you are an external observer, who can see things as what they really are without being emotionally influenced. Doing the same with yourself is not very easy, but a few minutes of good daily workout will surely help.

Translated by Laura Monti – Milan (Italy)

You need to create a self-consciousness center outside your body to act as an observer. With your mind, start to imagine that this center is inside a dot or a bead that is located outside you and above your head, is part of you, and is always with you. As you train this bead swells; as you manage to observe yourself from the outside, you also learn to observe your emotions, your frustrations, your biases, and to improve the aspects of your life to which you are often slave and subjected. This brings new solutions.

In fact, playing this "trick" will teach you to find solutions that you couldn't find for yourself, but would still have found for your imaginary friend. It is certainly not easy, or something you can strengthen, stabilize, and make effective within a month, but if you take it as a game, rather than as a job, it can give you valuable hints on your personality. Your self-consciousness and awareness center (enclosed in the imaginary bead located above your head) acts as your superconscious mind that you can identify and use, and is not vulnerable to your biases, your emotions, and your conditionings.

This is an oriental methodology, whose practitioners are masters to us in the west in terms of management of the mind and feelings. In fact, through globalization, some methodologies that used to be confined to certain parts of the eastern world are now also known and accessible in America and Europe.

Translated by Laura Monti – Milan (Italy)

We own our body. If I tell you to raise your arm and you want to, you can easily do so (unless you have physical disabilities). However, we are not as good at controlling our emotions, our fears, our apprehensions, our anxieties, our moods (all aspects that often influence and control us). This self-consciousness and awareness center allows you to detach yourself (with time and exercise) in such a way as to achieve a closer control of your mind.

Another method I want to suggest is to exploit the power of the unconscious and superconscious mind. When you have questions about your life and, specifically, about CH, consider them when you are about to fall asleep. It sometimes happens that, during the following day(s), your conscious mind magically comes up with the answers to your questions. The brain keeps working, it never stops, not even at night, while you sleep! Thus when you are half-asleep or just woke up (but in this case it is more difficult), ask yourself the questions you cannot answer consciously, and let your unconscious mind work on them. It has the answers.

If you have limiting defects – such as being inconsistent, having no self-confidence, not being determined, etc. – and soon end up with giving up your goals (e.g. simply going to the gym), you can also find a solution to these limits. This may be your characteristic, but you can change it if you know how to. Keep

Translated by Laura Monti – Milan (Italy)

repeating to yourself, in your conscious mind, whenever you can, hundreds of times a day. **"I am determined, I am consistent, I am self-confident."** This will start engraving the instruction contrary to your belief in your unconscious mind, thus generating a small synapse that you should strengthen by continuously repeating that positive statement. Our unconscious mind is "stupid" (meaning that it doesn't sort out true or false inputs, but only records them). If you know how, you can reset it through your conscious and intelligent mind.

Repeating this "new trick" for several months will convince your unconscious mind that you are consistent, and it will autonomously order you to be consistent. You just have to take action, when you know something and have a solution don't brood on it but take action, a smart action, and you will get your results! You don't need a great wisdom to transform yourself, you just have to keep "taking action."

It is not a matter of few days, this is wishful thinking, but in time you can do it. It means being proactive, not just passive, perhaps even scaling down some medications that affect you emotions or mood, cause anxiety, etc. They help too, but you are the most effective vehicle to transform your beast and much more. For sure, medications cannot change it, but they can help.

Two main factors are known today to program the unconscious mind by acting on the synapses: one is continuous repetition

Translated by Laura Monti – Milan (Italy)

over time (both mechanical/physical and mental thinking), the other is emotion (joy, happiness, fear, disappointment, suffering, anger, etc.). The emotional side is stronger, so it acts even without repetition.

The mind is much better known today, and world-famous coaches themselves (such as mental trainers) are the first to leverage upon this knowledge, so that we can understand and apply it to ourselves.

Partially simplifying the concept I wish to express, let us first consider that our head houses a conscious mind (the frontal lobe) that thinks, reasons, learns, calculates, and mostly lives in the past and in the future, and an unconscious mind that is always focused on the present and is programmed since our birth. The unconscious mind, as programmed in time, influences the body downstream to all the inputs it receives (environmental, emotional, relational, mechanical, and informational in a broad sense).

The conscious mind is intelligent, thinks, and is capable to make choices.

On the other hand, the unconscious mind is not intelligent, it is completely neutral. Somehow it can even be deemed stupid and, if poorly programmed, it has a self-destructive power, it doesn't

Translated by Laura Monti – Milan (Italy)

think and is not able to make choices, but it makes you act and often (in most cases) controls you!

In bytes (just to use a measurement unit), the conscious mind has an infinitely weaker operating power compared to the unconscious mind, which boasts an exponentially higher processing potential.

The unconscious mind acts as a real program and works regardless of right or wrong, good or bad, healthy or unhealthy. It acts/reacts according to how it was created in the course of the life of a human being. The unconscious mind may act either like a program designed for automated food distribution in a kennel (therefore to feed pets, something good), or like a program created to drop bombs and kill (something bad). Unlike the conscious mind, which is capable to decide and choose, it cannot decide, it is just enabled, and that's it.

Most of our being and our living is now known to be dictated more by our unconscious programming than by our will or by our control of the conscious one.

Unconscious programming may also help automation to enhance our skills by taking some jobs away from the conscious mind to entrust them to the unconscious mind, which can handle many more bytes. Here is a practical example: think about the first time you drove a car. Someone told your conscious mind what

Translated by Laura Monti – Milan (Italy)

you should do to drive: make adjustments — seat, rear-view mirror, side mirrors. Then ignite the engine either by setting it to neutral or pressing the clutch. At that point check that nothing hampers your way (nearing cars, pedestrians, motorcycles, bicycles, etc.) and gently release the clutch by pressing the accelerator. Who did it right the first time, without making the car choke or go off before coordinating the clutch and the accelerator? I think no one and, if someone did, it would be the exception that proves the rule! Having said that, every time you had to started your car and did your exercise to get it right, you had to think about it! You thought about it with your conscious mind based on the information you received from your instructor, your father, or a friend teaching you. Then, once you were moving, you had to change gear and at first you always had to think about it and you did it slowly; inside you, in your frontal mind, you repeated the instructions: I have to press the clutch, shift into second gear, then release the clutch while pressing down the accelerator. Repetition and training made you learn to do all this correctly. Now, by way of example, think whether, while doing this you would also be able to take a phone call, adjust your radio, take your jacket from the back seat, and look at that nice dog on the sidewalk!

While you were first learning to drive, your conscious mind was so busy it had to keep focused and alert to repeat the car driving

Translated by Laura Monti – Milan (Italy)

exercise correctly. It was so busy it couldn't do anything else and perhaps even generated such emotions as mild fear, anxiety and, to some people, physical reactions, such as sweating or tremor (depending on the psycho-emotional characteristics of each individual). Now move forward a few years and ask yourself whether, even after just three years, as you get into your car, you have to think about how hard you need to press the accelerator to start, how slowly you have to release the clutch, or that you have to press the clutch to change gear. We both know that the answer is no! You do everything automatically because you no longer use your conscious mind, but a program written in your unconscious mind generates synapses and makes you act automatically. You gave a program to your unconscious mind. With repetition you have trained your unconscious mind, which now works automatically and leaves your conscious mind free. Now, after several years driving, you drive without thinking and you can use your conscious mind for something else – to put on your favorite music, to take the CD, to take and light a cigarette, perhaps you take your hands off the steering wheel and hold it with your knee, have a casual chat with someone, or call your partner on the phone and even manage to argue with him/her brooding on what happened last night. And all the while you feel safe, no sweating and no anxiety.

Translated by Laura Monti – Milan (Italy)

In practice, the bytes of the conscious mind (which are more limited than those of the unconscious mind) that at first were so busy programming the unconscious mind, are now completely free to do other things because the task is automatically performed by the unconscious mind that, at the same time, does thousands of other things, most of which you are not even aware of!

This is how it works, but not because I say so! I only say what I learnt from those who are far more knowledgeable than me. If you dwell for a moment on what I said, you realize that this works on most things, not all though, that is, the unconscious mind is not only programmed through training and repetition. The process in the example, on the operation of the human body, is mechanical and similar to learning how to ride a bike, skateboarding, skating, or skiing – body functioning and communication between the conscious and the unconscious mind.

The only unconscious program that nature provides us from birth is the program for survival. This information comes from God and is also found in single-cell organisms.

In this respect our multi-cell body, made up of organs constituted by cells, each specializing in a specific task, does not differ from single-cell organisms. A cell can do either of two things, but never at the same time: fight/flee or feed, grow, and

Translated by Laura Monti – Milan (Italy)

reproduce itself. Any living being, from the amoeba to the cat to the human being, if under threat (therefore attacked by a highly stressful event), goes into the fight-or-flight mode and in that mode can neither take food, nor grow or reproduce itself. In human beings, programming for survival when facing a life threat is now known to cause a third reaction: not just fight or flight, but also stop. This is thoroughly explained in a nice book by Bruce Lipton, "The biology of beliefs."

Another natural macro and microscopic law that belongs to the "Whole" is the law of equilibrium: everything in nature tends to an equilibrium. Just think of the cosmic equilibrium of the solar system and of the planets' motion (which dates back to Kepler's physics), of atomic equilibrium, i.e. of how an atom is made, after the enlightening discoveries of Max Born: a neutron and a proton within a nucleus with electrons gravitating around. In fact ionization occurs to pursue the atom's energetic equilibrium. Let us set aside, for the moment, the concepts discovered by quantum physics that are likely to bring about a quantum leap in our evolution.

If we observe the microscopic or macroscopic aspects of nature, we always see it tends towards an equilibrium that is either energetic or functional. I think that the "Law of Equilibrium" is a "Law of Life," like that of the survival of all living beings.

Translated by Laura Monti – Milan (Italy)

Therefore, the unconscious mind also sets its priorities through the programming it receives during the life cycle of a human being. The main priority is the primordial programming we all share, aimed at survival.

Now, consider that pain and fear are both allies, because they send a warning sign or communicate a hazard that may put our survival at stake. All genetic programming for survival and the involuntary functioning of the human body (breathing, heartbeat, etc.) is inherent in our neuroendocrine system and basically belongs to the amygdalae and the hypothalamus. Its priority is to enable conditions/reactions, such as fight/flee/stop, which prevail over our will and the influence and decision-making power of the conscious mind. However, the conscious mind can always come into play and use awareness and decision-making, as well as specific exercises, to change the mechanisms triggered by the neuroendocrine system, which are linked – in this specific example – to a reaction for survival, and thus change our state from fight/flee/stop to feed/grow/reproduce yourself.

To make these difficult concepts clearer, I report an example of this function of our brain and of the relationship and influence between the conscious and unconscious mind in what is a non-pharmacological solution to address and then treat a disorder such as a "panic attack."

Translated by Laura Monti – Milan (Italy)

A panic attack is fear at its highest level. As I mentioned above, our unconscious mind can also respond to incorrect programming, which is detrimental to our health, and be activated, in response to the "programming of the Law of Survival," following a subsequent programming received from a life experience. It is both a repetitive and an emotional experiential programming.

I explain this with a real-life example.

A little girl about one year old sat in a car with her parents. The car was hit by a train while crossing the tracks. Before the collision, the train whistled for a long time. After the impact the parents died and the little girl survived. Of course that poor thing had no memory of the accident in her conscious mind, but her unconscious mind recorded the whole event in the amygdalae as a terrible traumatic experience to be afraid of and to react against in defense (fight/flee/stop). This severe trauma engaged all the 5 senses of the child in an environmental and physical association; it was incorporated in her brain (including the train's whistle) and recorded in her amygdalae, which are part of the neuroendocrine system responsible for enabling responses connected with and related to survival.

Over time this little girl grew up and became a teen-ager. During her adolescence she began to suffer from panic attacks that gradually got worse to the point they caused actual disability. In

Translated by Laura Monti – Milan (Italy)

addition to taking medications, the girl, by then a woman, had psychotherapy and regressive hypnosis sessions. Over time she discovered and became consciously aware that her panic attacks appeared every time her unconscious mind heard a sound/whistle similar to that of the train that killed her parents in the crash.

What happened after this new awareness of the conscious mind? When she happened to hear an acoustic trigger of a panic attack, the attack occurred (because, as mentioned above, the inputs of the survival program to the neuroendocrine system, which enable the fight/flee/stop reaction, prevail), but through gradual awareness and conscious reasoning, she managed to stop it. It was a hard and fruitless work at first, but over time she was able to stop her panic attacks faster, and was finally healed from this disorder, this unconscious disruptive health program.

This demonstrates that our unconscious programming can be influenced and changed (when negative or dysfunctional) to the benefit of our health.

Now I want you to dwell on another operation mode of memory in our brain in case, for example, of reactive depression, a disorder that is often a consequence of cluster headache.

Reactive depression is different from primary depression, which involves genetic issues affecting serotonin production.

Translated by Laura Monti – Milan (Italy)

Reactive depression occurs because of the influence of our biochemistry, due to a combination of sadness/negativity/suffering, emotionally induced by our conscious thinking.

I use this new example to make myself clearer. Someone that suffers a major bereavement (the death of a parent, a child, or a brother) is generally sad and ailing, and his or her mood falls into depression. Generally these people should not be prescribed medications acting on brain biochemistry, because after a while, once they accept the tragedy, their balance is spontaneously restored, and depression subsides. However, in some individuals that fail to overcome their bereavement and keep brooding on it, the feelings of sorrow and sadness are self-fueled and their depression does not subside. According to science, if such depression does not subside within, on average, three months, antidepressants may be required to help influence brain biochemistry. Why does this happen? Because the functioning of our brain (thinking, emotions, spirit, conscious mind, and unconscious mind) can become dysfunctional. If protracted in time, a faulty biochemistry (of an unhealthy kind) induced by conscious thinking is recorded in our brain as normal functioning and stored. The brain actually memorizes that this altered biochemistry is the norm and repeats it as the norm, even if it is no longer induced by thought. This is where reactive depression starts as a true illness, generated by the inability to overcome

Translated by Laura Monti – Milan (Italy)

bereavement. Today, science demonstrates that there are two ways out of this problem: one relies on antidepressants to restore the biochemical balance artificially; they are taken for a reasonable period of time to restore the appropriate biochemistry in the inner memory (as it was previously) and then, once this is achieved, they are gradually phased out to give time to the brain to take action to keep the new stored balance.

The other option is a so-called "re-education" with an experienced educator. Re-education is focused on the conscious mind, on the thoughts that trigger emotions, and on the body's physical action/reaction. If well re-educated, the individual recovers from reactive depression by modifying brain biochemistry through the emotional power released by the conscious mind.

Don't get me wrong, though. With the above, I am not claiming that CH is a psychiatric condition.

However, that type of illness and pain has actually a significant impact on our psyche and can generate consequential co-morbidities, including reactive depression or panic attacks. This is why I gave these two examples. I could give many others, but that is not my purpose. My purpose is to tell you things that maybe you didn't know and that can support you and help you cope with all the implications of your beast and design strategies

Translated by Laura Monti – Milan (Italy)

that you can rely upon to trigger a potential transformation towards greater well-being or a lesser malaise.

Indeed, your beast involves the neuroendocrine system (as scientifically demonstrated by German researchers) that, as mentioned, can be partially impacted. That reactive depression is a consequence of CH is not important; what is important is that it is also a promoter. Thus, when I say you have to "wear it down", I also mean you have to stop the self-promoting cycle that is sometimes observed in severe CH.

In this book I am only trying to share with you all the self-help weapons that may be useful, all my knowledge that I believe, hope, and trust you can leverage upon to understand and transform your beast for the sole purpose of your well-being.

FRIENDS, FAMILY, DOCTORS, SCHOLARS

Hello, who are you? Are you a friend of a CH sufferer, or perhaps a co-worker? Are you a family member, a parent, a partner, or a spouse? Are you a doctor or a scholar wishing to specialize in neurology or headaches?

Well, if you belong to one of the above groups I think this book can be of great help for you too, something that can give you ideas for action, tell you more about this severe illness, offer you

Translated by Laura Monti – Milan (Italy)

suggestions to interact with a CH sufferer, give you personal hints to think about this nasty beast – in short, I hope and trust it will help you too!

Dear friend or co-worker, even if unconsciously, you can often be a source of further anger or pain for the CH sufferer. This certainly doesn't happen out of malice, but only because of your poor knowledge of the disease or poor empathy, sometimes even out of mere flippancy or selfishness.

Being a friend of a CH sufferer, one that forces you to share his or her suffering when you go out together, that doesn't let you enjoy a full evening out (for a pizza, a walk, dancing, a swim, or anything else), is certainly not easy or enjoyable. This sometimes leads to a kind of annoyance that spontaneously makes you say things that hurt your friend, like "Shit, what a drag," "Cut it short and take an Advil®," "Alright, next time I'll go in Mark's (or any other friend's) car, at least I'll be sure I can stay out," "You can't go on complaining about your headache," "Come on now, you want to go home for a mere headache, I'm not coming with you anymore," "A headache again... get treated," "Enough with that, do you want me to have a headache too?" "If you feel cold, I think it's because you are wearing nothing warm! I think it's because you ate too much! I think it's because you didn't have enough sleep! I think... I think... I think!"

Translated by Laura Monti – Milan (Italy)

As I said, being a friend or a co-worker of a CH sufferer and share part of his or her life "is certainly not easy or enjoyable" for you, but did you ever ask yourself what does it mean to them? Did you ever get sympathetically in their shoes? **If you're a true friend, do it!** The life of a CH sufferer is an ordeal and friends are there to share pleasant moments, but also to rely upon at times of trouble. Nurturing a true friendship also means giving something up and knowing how to make the right choices for the sake of your friend. **What do you think is more valuable: a pleasant night out or "true friendship"?** Look, life is a continuous change, a continuous transformation, and perhaps one day your roles will be reversed and you will be the one in need of a true friend, someone by your side to help you... not to leave you behind or attack you!

Diminishing the trouble of an upcoming CH attack and suggesting to take a painkiller arouses a sufferer's anger and forces him or her to explain things they already explained before, so it means feeding the attack then, and the beast in time. Be a true friend, accept the situation and stand by until they recover from the attack. If it is an excruciating attack and they have no medications with them, take them to an ER, explain their case to the doctors, and ask them to skip the waiting list and give him a shot of sumatriptan right away.

Translated by Laura Monti – Milan (Italy)

Statements like "I think..." are inappropriate. If it is CH, that's it, there is no "I think"; the "I think" only pisses your friend off, and forces him or her to provide exhaustive explanations right when the attack is rising. By doing so, you hurt them!

If you are a true friend of a CH sufferer you have to acknowledge your friend's tragedy and provide psychological support, if necessary proactively. A friend of a guy with epilepsy normally does not tell him off when he has an attack; if he is knowledgeable, he stands by him and tries to prevent him from getting hurt or swallowing his tongue, but things are often different for CH sufferers! Why? I believe it is because of poor knowledge of the illness, which is less visible and often associated with common headache, but in truth an attack is a severe crisis that involves the whole being. It is not just expressed with pain, but also with other important neurovegetative and psychological signs. **If you are a friend of a CH sufferer, learn about the disease and try to help him or her, or you wouldn't be a friend. Ask yourself!**

When CH sufferers beat around the bush with their illness, it's because they need to speak, to pour out their sorrow, they seek understanding, they seek your friendship. Let them speak and humor them. If they become too verbose, explain that perhaps it is bad for them to continue to keep this thought alive, generating negative emotions and feeding the beast. Kindly suggest them to

Translated by Laura Monti – Milan (Italy)

try to think about it only when they are suffering for an attack, otherwise to pretend they didn't have CH. This is somehow the concept I discussed in previous chapter: open and close the parenthesis when you suffer and then try not to continue to keep your illness "alive" in thoughts. This is the greatest help you can give a CH sufferer.

Remember, if you are a friend, you must be a "true friend"!

I try to make you understand what a CH sufferer experiences when faced with these situations. Riccardo Pentenero, the first CH sufferer I met and with whom I founded OUCH Italy, together with others, was very good at using the internet and websites. The first website on CH he created had a section dedicated to his colleagues at work, who tended to diminish his illness and claimed he didn't want to work. Well, the website included a section on his advice to other CH sufferers when facing such attitude in their colleagues. The advice was expressed with a drawing: **a death wish for the damned colleague!** This was a strong emotional expression of Riccardo. Just imagine the level to which his unsympathetic colleagues raised his anger.

With the family or partner it gets even more complicated. Intimate relations are stronger and love tends to be greater. The big problem is that a family member, whether a parent or a partner, may often need psychological support to live with a CH sufferer, particularly if chronic. Their involvement can be so

Translated by Laura Monti – Milan (Italy)

frequent, so close, and so strong as to cause them suffering in turn. Advice to try to reduce one's empathy can be obtained from a specialized psychologist dealing with suffering. I don't mean that the partner or parent has psychological problems, but that such involvement in the suffering of a loved one may have two critical outcomes: one is their own suffering and need for help (not physical, but psychological suffering), and the other is something like the burnout syndrome, often observed in physicians and nurses that take care of patients with chronic and degenerative diseases. It is a sort of emotional stress-related exhaustion.

In the vast majority of cases, family members go to extremes to help, but most of the times they have no hints, they do something and see it doesn't work, stand by while their dear one suffers and are sent away, face and suffer an anger that is not for them, but is generated in the CH sufferer that turns against them, witness hardly tolerable situations… and they are not professional medical practitioners or nurses, trained to cope with these cases.

In the burnout syndrome, specialized physicians or nurses, who are also trained to deal with patient suffering and care, often lose self-confidence and feel they are not up to the ordeal. Hence one of the causes of the onset of the syndrome.

Translated by Laura Monti – Milan (Italy)

Let us now imagine similar situations involving ordinary people, such as family members whose job is other than in the medical field and who receive no support, do not speak with psychologists to receive assistance to address these challenges. I think illnesses like the burnout syndrome should certainly be taken seriously.

These points are of great importance, even if still hardly considered. Family members challenged with a chronic CH sufferer in the family that necessarily affects their life must be conscious and aware of the situation and find the courage to seek help to deal with it in the broadest sense. **Only if they are comfortable, cool, and detached with respect to the extreme suffering of their beloved, will they be able to help him or her.**

Now let's see how. As mentioned, at first they should take care of themselves and learn how to manage their emotional and psychological attitude. Most aspects of the relation with CH sufferers should be studied over time and discussed with them. Let me give you a personal practical example that I found to be different in other CH sufferers. When an attack is about to arise, I notice even before I feel the pain. At that stage, if my partner pampers me, scratches my head, or lightly touches my back, neck, or other sensitive points, I feel utmost pleasure because at those times I am more sensitive than usual, and the attack may even subside. On the other hand, during an acute attack I want

Translated by Laura Monti – Milan (Italy)

to be alone, I don't want anyone to see me, I even tend to be rude to people if they insist on remaining close to me. Other CH sufferers can be annoying in the pre-attack phase, and do not tolerate physical contact. Others yet, during the attack, feel scared to the extent that they want to have someone near rather than be alone. It is a very subjective relational aspect that needs to be understood and investigated to decide what to do.

Practical hints in terms of support and assistance can help deal with the situation. For example, remind the CH sufferer to always record each event in a headache diary, in order to give the neurologist objective feedback during follow-up checks. Sometimes the sufferer can hardly be objective and consistent. Here is some of my experience before I started to write an accurate diary. At first, when my CH was episodic, if I saw the neurologist for a check while deep in a cluster, with daily attacks for maybe a month, I was so exhausted that I tended to report a longer time frame, since I hadn't taken notes and did not remember when it had started. A whole month with the attacks seemed to me much longer, and that's why I made inaccurate reports. If asked when it had started, I might answer a couple of months before. On the other hand, when my CH became chronic, with attacks throughout the year for years, I occasionally happened to have none for two or three days. In that case, if those that knew me and knew I suffered from CH asked me "How are you?", I answered "Very well, thank-you", because at

Translated by Laura Monti – Milan (Italy)

that moment I felt as strong as a lion. Indeed, I wasn't well at all, I still felt very bad in terms of headache, because the day after I could very well revert to three or four daily attacks and suffer excruciatingly. Therefore, the emotional state of a CH sufferer that remembers exactly how he or she did in, say, the last three months, which is a customary term for follow-up checks, influences and affects the objectiveness of the answers. **This makes it critical to keep and regularly update a headache diary, a task that could be shared with family members wishing to help their loved one.**

Other objective practical approaches that can be of help in the family include recording whether the intake of certain foods triggers an attack. CH attacks often occur at night, but also during the day. If they don't always happen at the same time during the day, and sometimes they do after meals, it is good to record what you had, and then check over time whether a specific food is a trigger.

You can also try to remind the CH sufferer to drink a lot of water, if he or she doesn't already do so, because it helps. Headache sufferers tend to drink very little.

You can help them remember to take their pills, perhaps buying one of those pill holders that produce an acoustic warning at the scheduled time.

Translated by Laura Monti – Milan (Italy)

It is also very important to listen to the CH sufferer, who needs to discharge his or her anger. Make them cry so that they pour out some of their emotion and stress (I tended to keep back tears, I kept everything within), encourage them, keep their hope alive, because emotions are very important and many sufferers tend to be overwhelmed by discomfort and, if so, they feed the beast.

Follow your loved one by lovingly making him or her do whatever it takes to take care of their health and, most of all, to reduce stressful events.

If they tend to oversleep on Saturdays and Sundays or during the holidays, wake them up gently and lovingly because, as explained above, changing from little resting and great stress to full rest and relaxation is something that tends to worsen or trigger CH.

While this chapter could provide an even broader range of guidelines for family members, spouses, or parents, I think that reading this book may have given you so much food for thought and so much new knowledge that you can leverage upon. Do not just read the book, but also keep up to date by attending some national and international forums to learn more and more.

Don't forget to encourage your family member with CH to attend patient forums, if he or she doesn't already – some tend to withdraw, by their temperament or reactivity. Encouraging them

Translated by Laura Monti – Milan (Italy)

to make friends with others that suffer from the same disease is a kind of psychological therapy, as I noticed in 95% of the cases I observed over ten years in the association.

Your involvement, your action, and your participation are very important, but don't forget about yourself: **first take care of the negative emotional impact you may experience, in order to be steady and reliable, because being able to help requires your being in good health.**

And here we come to a crucial and more delicate point: the children of CH sufferers. When a CH sufferer has a child, he or she should also think about protecting such child. The younger the child, the greater the protection needed. Over time he or she should then be made gradually aware of mum's or dad's illness. The frontal cortex of a child is not fully developed, there is no brain "programming" and life is mainly made of feelings and emotions. As they grow up, they start to know and understand about life, the world, and their surroundings, they learn to distinguish between good and bad, joy and pain, etc. Emotional education is crucial in children. I am not a child psychologist and am not very sure about the most appropriate approaches. I'm just saying this out of common sense.

In the first months/years of life, I would keep the child away from his or her parent's suffering because, as I said, children have feelings and emotions, even if their cognitive

Translated by Laura Monti – Milan (Italy)

understanding is still underdeveloped. They even have some "sixth sense," which then (generally) fades away as they grow up, so that they can sense that mum is suffering even from a distance. Having said that, **I think it's wrong to have them see their parent suffer a CH crisis.** I also think that, over time, they should be talked to gently and progressively, so that they know that mum or dad feels pain at certain times of the day. "Do you remember? It's like when you burned your finger, or fell and scratched your knees." In short, give them simple examples that they can understand. This may help them understand why mum or dad sometimes lock themselves away, or why they hear them moan. Later on, of course, more accurate explanations can be provided, but I don't think I should mention a right age at which the different steps towards the truth can be made. **However, I think I can recommend seeking family counseling or specialist child psychology support to receive the best possible advice.**

In my experience I noticed a kind of fear in my eldest daughter when she saw me suffer during and after an attack, and I think I wasn't able to handle this aspect in the right way. The mere thought arouses regret, because I should have thought about it earlier and taken care of prevention.

I now wish to focus on what is one of the most important factors for the treatment of a CH sufferer: the doctor in the broadest sense, either a general practitioner or a specialist (neurologist),

Translated by Laura Monti – Milan (Italy)

but also an undergraduate wishing to specialize in the field of headaches.

I first wish to point out that in the past history of the CH sufferers I dealt with, as well as in my own personal experience, it took years and several incorrect treatments before we could obtain a correct diagnosis and a well-designed therapeutic approach. Cluster headache is, indeed, easy to diagnose, its characteristics are quite easy to identify. In the past, part of the misdiagnoses could be due to poor knowledge of the specific illness, which was then approached inappropriately.

The main problem is that this mistake, if extended in time, can make CH even worse if inadequate medications are used. Consider that even the overuse of appropriate symptomatic medications like sumatriptan can result into triptan intoxication that feeds the beast. Therefore, when facing this condition, a wise specialist would often recommend hospitalization for blood washing. As you can imagine, it is even worse if you take medications that are not specifically indicated for CH. As a hint to general practitioners, I recommend that they first inquire about cluster headache and, if in doubt, refer the patient to an accredited headache center without making attempts upon their own initiative because, even if made with the best intentions, they can do more harm than good.

Translated by Laura Monti – Milan (Italy)

However, in headache centers or in neurological units in general you can face contradictions due to a "sick system" that is more focused on making money for the "facility" than on helping those that suffer. This refers to the time slots in protocols, which are often too small to allow a careful examination. For example, an examination should last 15 to 20 minutes, but how can a diligent doctor get to know and understand a patient, ask the necessary questions, provide the appropriate diagnosis, reassure and gain the patient's confidence in such a short time? The doctor-patient relation is crucial for treatment, because it involves the psychological sphere, the hope that the doctor should instill, which is part of a placebo effect that always plays a role and, last but not least, the patient's trust in the neurologist. I think all these aspects are of great importance, as much as the appropriate medications and doses prescribed by the specialist from time to time to help the patient. You could see that CH is, indeed, easy to diagnose by its symptoms, but it is also extremely subjective. This is why it is so important to investigate the patient in all respects (not just his or her symptoms).

CH sufferers are quite peculiar individuals. They usually need to talk, to pour out their emotions, to understand that all their CH-related disorders are connected with CH and not stand-alone. These include sleep and mood disorders, neurovegetative and psychological ones that may occur over time, such as anxiety, potential or actual reactive depression, or panic. I don't mean

Translated by Laura Monti – Milan (Italy)

that a neurologist dealing with cluster headache should also act as a psychologist (in fact, in some cases, he or she may refer a CH sufferer to a psychologist), but some basic psychologist's skills are required to take the right approach to patients.

I touched upon this aspect because I think it is important to encourage neurologists to become our allies, to really want to help us, to give us their own mind on this aspect, as well as to make ethically professional, albeit uncomfortable choices against the "System."

In fact, the "Hippocratic Oath" is not intended to produce more money for the facility that employs them! Or is it?

"The Hippocratic Oath - Modern Text"

Aware of the importance and solemnity of the act I perform and the commitment I make,

I SWEAR:

- *to exercise medicine in freedom and independence of judgment and conduct;*

- *to pursue the defense of life, the protection of man's physical and mental health and the relief of suffering, which I will inspire with responsibility and constant scientific, cultural and social commitment, every one of my professional actions as exclusive goals;*

- *to never perform acts suitable to deliberately cause the death of a patient;*

- *to abide by my ethical principles of human solidarity, against which, in respect of life and of the person, I will never use my knowledge;*

- to perform my work with diligence, skill and prudence according to knowledge and conscience and observing the deontological norms that regulate the practice of medicine and the juridical ones which do not conflict with the purposes of my profession;

- to entrust my reputation exclusively to my professional skills and moral qualities;

- to avoid, even outside of professional practice, any act and behavior that may damage the prestige and dignity of the profession;

- to respect colleagues even in the event of conflicting opinions;

- to treat all my patients with equal care and commitment regardless of the feelings they inspire me and regardless of any difference in race, religion, nationality, social condition and political ideology;

- to provide emergency assistance to any patient who needs it and to put me in the service of the competent authority in the event of a public disaster;

- to respect and facilitate in any case the right of the patient to the free choice of his doctor, taking into account that the relationship between doctor and patient is based on trust and in any case on mutual respect;

- to observe the secret of everything that is confided to me, that I see or have seen, understood or sensed in the exercise of my profession or because of my state.

An appropriate medical examination should last, for some people, 20 minutes, for others 90 minutes. There is no standard time based on management procedures, but it is up to a wise neurologist to decide.

Doctor, what does your conscience suggest you to do in your often tough environment? Because you have a soul, a

Translated by Laura Monti – Milan (Italy)

conscience, and the role you play in society is too important to be confined to mere financial income! This is just my opinion and I don't mean to be abusive, but **sometimes, if I just think about it, in this frantic life imposed on us by the "System," this one can be a genuine and improving approach.**

Another aspect of cluster headache I would like neurologists to consider and think about is the need to grant a **"fast track for checks."**

In the past, I happened to be told I had to wait several months before I could get an appointment at a hospital headache center via the public healthcare system. **This is unsustainable for CH sufferers!**

Nowadays, an efficient organization is in place at some headache centers; waiting lists are not too long and you can get an appointment within a very short time, but this only happens at some advanced facilities. On the other hand, neurologists should promote this by adequately raising the awareness of decision-makers in this respect – whether the head physician or the health director. It is certainly a very important issue to be addressed and amended.

I would also like to encourage doctors to establish a two-way relationship with their patients, something that doesn't happen in some cases.

Translated by Laura Monti – Milan (Italy)

It is also important to keep constantly in touch with the patient, also while implementing a new therapy, to provide a step-by-step feedback (perhaps just via the e-mail) that can make a difference and to make any adjustments to the current therapy. I say this because sometimes, upon follow-up checks, I was prescribed a new medication and the next check was scheduled after three months, without establishing an open communication channel. **This approach always failed!**

I believe that reading this book, which originates from my personal experience in the field developed in a non-scientific, yet definitely experiential position, can also help doctors and scientists that wish to actually understand how someone that suffers from this goddamn disease lives. I also hope and trust it will inspire those that take a non-pharmacological approach to the treatment of CH. I wish to encourage neurologists to take a broader approach to CH, by which they can achieve more satisfactory results by recommending CH sufferers to "wear down" their illness, as discussed on the previous pages; encourage them to come out of their psychological confinement and attend the forums dedicated to CH to share their position and meet peers; refer those in need to psychological support in order to learn to live with pain and to accept their illness because, at psychological level, they tend to deny being sick, they tend to struggle against pain, to stiffen, to develop anger, reactivity, self-harm. When facing strong attacks, most people find themselves knocking their head against the wall, losing their temper.

I think most CH sufferers also need to be "educated" on their illness, on how to manage stress, on how to discharge, counter, mitigate it. This can be achieved in several ways, including dietary antioxidant supplementing, sports, but not too much, resting, meditation, yoga, mindfulness, psychological support, psychiatric support, emotional support, spiritual education, assertive attitude education, etc.

This more holistic approach to the illness is also intended to stimulate the patient's proactive attitude by removing the risk of taking a mere passive stance and developing medical-pharmacological dependence that hampers a potentially positive outcome.

I encourage you to use all the weapons at your disposal, because ultimately what matters is to achieve an improvement, beat CH, or reduce suffering, rather than know for sure which weapon was most effective.

Translated by Laura Monti – Milan (Italy)

CONCLUSION

Here we come to the conclusion of my book dedicated to you. If I had to summarize all the above in few words, no matter how hard it would be, I would say that **the beast is certainly one of the worst life companions you could have** – sometimes weakening, sometimes disabling, sometimes overwhelming, because it cancels your life, your personality, in order to be the only one there to overwhelm you like a stormy sea.

I provided a number of definitions because, indeed, CH is not always the same from an individual to the next, as well as for the same individual in the course of its development. This is shown by the cluster of episodic sufferers: it begins with almost tolerable attacks, which increase in intensity over time until they reach their climax and then decrease and subside.

Chronic CH has a different pattern: the attacks can be of variable intensity, but the bad thing is that they continue throughout your life. Like a drop of water that always falls on the same point and digs a hole in a rock, chronic CH can destroy the strongest of men. It is a strange illness, a unique illness, and I think that we CH sufferers are also unique people. It is an illness that is rooted in us, an illness that belongs to us but, as such, I believe it is also

Translated by Laura Monti – Milan (Italy)

within our capability to influence, both in a positive and in a negative way.

The negative way is the most spontaneous, almost automated, because your sadness arises spontaneously, you fall into depression spontaneously, you get mad at life spontaneously, you continue to think spontaneously, your fear arises spontaneously, and you condition your existence spontaneously. This spontaneity feeds the spiral into which you fall when you are hit by this illness.

In a positive way, however, it is much more difficult to interact with it, because it requires knowledge, willpower, persistence, constancy, and the application of techniques and methodologies repeated over again. Just like a drug that at some point in your CH was ineffective but may become effective if tried again, the techniques and approaches I described in the book can also be ineffective sometimes and effective some other times, and vice versa. While this is somewhat daunting, with the strength you have developed to endure your beast, you will surely manage.

I would say spontaneously that the first thing you should do now is to read the whole book once, then read it again and highlight the **key concepts** to start drafting a **voluntary action and counteraction plan.** This is a real job that implies drafting a do's and don'ts list, including drug and non-drug approaches, and recording the benefits or failures you experience from time to

Translated by Laura Monti – Milan (Italy)

time. Writing down things is fundamental, because the mind plays bad tricks when it comes to thinking about the pain that you have suffered.

When should you do that? Now, start now, right now, don't wait!

As a chronic sufferer, if I occasionally spent three days without attacks and someone asked me how I was, I answered "I'm fine, I feel as strong as a lion", but that wasn't true because CH was only granting me a few days of respite. Similarly, when you are sick and are asked how you feel, the answer is often, "I always have this damn headache," but this is not true either, you don't <u>always</u> have attacks on a 24-hour basis. That is why **you should learn how to open and close a parenthesis in your mind during each attack,** to avoid to drag it around all day long, at psychological level. This is why you need to write a diary for each event you face, because those will be real facts, rather than the mental distortion you experience at such hard times.

Once you have designed a counteraction plan to transform your beast, you must be more persistent than the cluster itself. You must implement your plan as spontaneously as you can, in the way it is designed in your mind, because **there cannot be two equal plans**. It must be customized according to your specific condition. **It is useful that you find a neurologist to plan your counterattack together,** because it must include medications, but remember it should "not be based on medications only " and

Translated by Laura Monti – Milan (Italy)

you must be a proactive player, not a passive patient of the doctor.

You should not be a "patient," not least because those who suffer so much from CH have more than exhausted their patience – the doctor (if anything) must be patient with us!

The most significant take-home message I wish to give you is my story. As I mentioned, my CH gradually developed into a chronic drug-resistant form, which is probably the worst case you can experience with the beast. I turned to the best doctors and coaches, I sought approaches out of official medicine, as well as out of medicine itself, and even failed with the proposed approach of Deep Brain Stimulation (inserting an electrode in my brain, when alert, to act as a stimulator on the hypothalamus).

I didn't give up, I went on "crawling on my elbows" but didn't give up. I studied, I got in touch with other CH sufferers to identify any common traits, I discovered new approaches and, partly out of determination and partly by chance, my beast began its transformation. I never knew about other cases like mine, I only heard about improvements or remissions with old age, but it is not my case, I was not that old when the beast began to surrender!

This is something significant I wish to share with you as a CH sufferer and with the family members you live with, any doctors

Translated by Laura Monti – Milan (Italy)

that wish to approach our problem sympathetically, any scientists that wish to study CH more thoroughly, and any undergraduates that wish to become neurologists specializing in headaches. This is why I laid my soul bare, so that the significance of my story can be of help to others.

I think I gave as much as I could to this subject and this issue that radically changed and affected my life and, as you can see, you can win. If I succeeded, you can also manage to transform your beast from an aggressive lion to a meek dog. Sometimes you will feel discouraged and defeated, but the only thing that matters is that **when you fall, you get up and continue on your way.** The road will be long, perhaps arduous, but step by step, sooner or later, you'll get to your destination. You must never give up, you must be strong, draw strength from yourself and from others, and ask nature to give you such strength – you will get it.

Imagine that you have already achieved your goal, despite the hard work ahead of you, and never get discouraged. Keep repeating to yourself, whenever you can – you have to do it every moment and every day of your life, like a mantra - "**I'm stronger**, I'm stronger, I'm stronger." Stick this concept deep into your unconscious mind, and the stronger will win. You must want it, remember **"If you want, you can."**

Translated by Laura Monti – Milan (Italy)

That's all folks. I wish you all the best and I convey my "quantum" strength to you, but I'll leave you with a question: **If I made it, why shouldn't you?**

I'M HERE, I'M BY YOUR SIDE! Goodbye.

Davide Luca Schiantarelli

Translated by Laura Monti – Milan (Italy)

DISCLAIMER

I, Davide Schiantarelli, am a cluster headache sufferer, and I am not a doctor.

As I explained in the book, I have lived with this serious disease and have dealt with it both scientifically and not. I have studied some areas and aspects of medicine, I have founded a no-profit association dedicated to cluster headache sufferers and have met many sufferers in order to carry out my own research aimed at understanding the causes, the common traits of sufferers, and anything useful to mitigate our suffering.

However, my book **is not and should not be intended as a scientific journal**, as I have neither the qualifications nor the authority to write one.

The book contains explanations of drug-related aspects, also mentioning symptomatic medications for the prophylactic treatment of cluster headache with the corresponding benefits and drawbacks. While that part of the book was reviewed by a neurologist specializing in headaches, I do not intend in any way whatsoever to suggest or recommend prescription drugs that are absolutely and necessarily subject to the sole responsibility of those that have the relevant scientific and legal competence.

Translated by Laura Monti – Milan (Italy)

What I wrote is pure information. I also release the neurologist mentioned in the book from any and all liabilities for my assertions, even if shared thereby.

All the other descriptions of non-pharmacological aspects, whether related to the mentioned medications, to the use of water and oxygen, to nutrition, to the holistic vision, or to psychological aspects, are pure information I wish to share as a result of my work on the subject, and I don't want them to be taken as absolute certainties. I also take no liability whatsoever for any uses and applications attempted without the consent of a physician, where legally required.

Indeed, I share everything I know to try and help others, whether sufferers, family members of sufferers, or researchers on cluster headache, but I don't want to and cannot be intended as a physician, because I am not.

While most of my past insights were then confirmed by the scientific community, all the assumptions, hypotheses, or information I have published have no scientific value to date. However, I hope and trust that perhaps, in the future, they will play a role as a starting point for new investigations and research by the scientific community.

Translated by Laura Monti – Milan (Italy)

I inform seriously and honestly, then each individual is responsible for his or her own choices and decisions.

Translated by Laura Monti – Milan (Italy)

Printed in Great Britain
by Amazon